Philippine Resins, Gums, Seed Oils, and Essential Oils

By Augustus P. West, Ph. D.,

Professor of Chemistry, University of the Philippines

and

William H. Brown, Ph. D.,

Chief, Division of Investigation, Bureau of Forestry; Professor of Botany, University of the Philippines; and Plant Physiologist, Bureau of Science

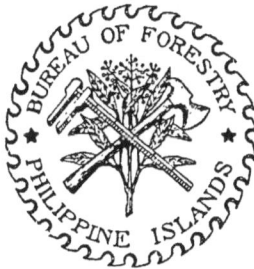

Department of Agriculture and Natural Resources
Bureau of Forestry

Bulletin No. 20

Arthur F. Fischer, Director of Forestry

British Library Cataloguing-in-Publication Data
A catalogue record for this book is available from the
British Library

Essential Oils

Essential oils are also known as volatile oils, ethereal oils, aetherolea, or simply as the 'oil of' the plant from which they are extracted, such as the oil of clove. An oil is 'essential' in the sense that it contains the characteristic fragrance of the plant that it is taken from. Essential oils do not form a distinctive category for any medicinal, pharmacological, or culinary purpose - and they are not essential for health, although they have been used medicinally in history. Although some are suspicious or dismissive towards the use of essential oils in healthcare or pharmacology, essential oils retain considerable popular use, partly in fringe medicine and partly in popular remedies. Therefore it is difficult to obtain reliable references concerning their pharmacological merits.

Medicinal applications proposed by those who sell or use medical oils range from skin treatments to remedies from cancer - and are generally based on historical efficacy. Having said this, some essential oils such as those of juniper and agathosma are valued for their diuretic effects. Other oils, such as clove oil or eugenol were popular for many hundreds of years in dentistry and as antiseptics and local anaesthetics. However as the use of essential oils has declined in evidence based medicine, older text-books are frequently our only sources for information!   Modern works are less inclined to generalise; rather than referring to 'essential oils' as a class at all, they prefer to discuss specific compounds, such as methyl salicylate, rather than 'oil of wintergreen.'

Nevertheless, interest in essential oils has considerably revived in recent decades, with the popularity of aromatherapy, alternative health stores and massage. Generally, the oils are volatized or diluted with a carrier oil to be used in massage, or diffused in the air by a nebulizer, heated over a candle flame, or burned as incense. Their usage goes way back, and the earliest recorded mention of such methods used to produce essential oils was made by Ibn al-Baitar (1188-1248), an Andalusian physician, pharmacist and chemist. Different oils were claimed to have differing properties; some to have an uplifting and energizing effect on the mind such as grapefruit and jasmine, whilst others such as rose lavender have a reputation as de-stressing and relaxing - and also, usefully, as an insect repellent.

The oils themselves are usually extracted by 'distillation', often by using steam -but some other processes include 'expression' or 'solvent extraction'. Distillation involves raw plant material (be that flowers, leaves, wood, bark, roots, seeds or peel) put into an alembic (distillation apparatus) over water. As the water is heated, the steam passes through the plant material, vaporizing the volatile compounds. The vapours flow through a coil, where they condense back to liquid, which is then collected in the receiving vessel. 'Expression' differs in that it usually merely uses a mechanical or cold press to extract the oil. Most citrus peel oils are made in this way, and due to the relatively large quantities of oil in citrus peel and low cost to grow and harvest the raw materials, citrus-fruit oils are cheaper than most other essential oils. 'Solvent extraction' is perhaps the most difficult of the three methods, and is generally used for flowers, which contain too little volatile oil to undergo expression. Instead, a solvent such as hexane or supercritical carbon dioxide is used to extract the oils.

These techniques have allowed essential oils to be used in all manner of products; from perfumes to cosmetics, soaps - and as flavourings for food and drinks as well as adding scent to incense and household cleaning products. The science, history and folkloric tradition of essential oils is incredibly fascinating - and a still much debated area. We hope the reader is inspired by this book to find out more.

CONTENTS

3

ILLUSTRATIONS

7

PREFACE

For a number of years there has been in the Philippines considerable trade in the two resins, Manila copal or almaciga * and Manila elemi or brea blanca (Span., "white pitch"). The other resinous products of the Philippines have been used only to a very limited extent, while until recently there has been little commerce in Philippine oils other than ilang-ilang.

Copra, which is the dried meat of the coconut and the source of the coconut oil of commerce, was formerly shipped from the Philippines in large quantities. Of late, however, there has been an extensive development of the coconut-oil industry in the Archipelago, a number of oil mills having been established in Manila and other parts of the Islands. Consequently, coconut oil is now expressed from the copra in Philippine oil mills and exported to other countries. The local commercial activities in this industry have been greatly accelerated by conditions due to the recent world conflict.

This development of the coconut-oil industry has naturally led to a greatly increased interest in other oils and similar products; and so it seems fitting at this time to present a bulletin giving a short account of oils and resins which are the basis of commercial industries or which offer promising possibilities. From the discussions given in the introduction and in connection with the various species, it will be seen that a number of industries could be profitably developed, and that there are other new ones which are worthy of serious consideration.

In discussing the various species of plants, we have used the following system: On the left of the page is given the scientific name, and on the right the local name adopted as official by the Bureau of Forestry. A list of local names in the various dialects follows. The first part of the discussion takes up the general uses and importance of the products concerned. This is succeeded by a more technical description of the products, after

---

* The Spanish name almaciga which is properly the equivalent of the English gum mastic (the product of *Pistachia lentiscus*) was incorrectly applied by the Spaniards in the Philippines to the resin of *Agathis alba*, a coniferous tree, and has become the commercial name, throughout the Islands, of the resin known in Europe and America as Manila copal.

which a description of the species is given, followed by a short account of its distribution and abundance. The local names are very convenient as assisting in the identification of the species, but are by no means infallible guides. It is believed, however, that by use of the local names, descriptions, and figures, it will be possible in most cases to identify the various species.

In preparing this bulletin, the writers have received valuable assistance from many sources, but particularly from Mr. E. D. Merrill, Director of the Bureau of Science, and Mr. E. E. Schneider, wood expert of the Bureau of Forestry. The native names have been revised by Mr. Schneider, who is conversant with several Philippine dialects, and who has taken great interest in the proper spelling of local names of Philippine plants. The original drawings were made under the direction of Mr. J. K. Santos by Messrs. F. de la Costa, P. C. Cagampan, J. Pascasio, S. Calusin, and Miss Maria Pastrana.

The writers are indebted to the Bureau of Science for the cuts used for figures 1, 18, 26, 27, 29, 31, 33, 36, 37, 60, and 62; to the Bureau of Education for figures 51 and 59; and to the Bureau of Agriculture for figure 53.

AUGUSTUS P. WEST.
WILLIAM H. BROWN.

PHILIPPINE RESINS, GUMS, SEED OILS, AND ESSENTIAL OILS

By Augustus P. West and William H. Brown

INTRODUCTION

The Philippine forests contain a large number of trees and other plants which produce seed oils, essential oils, resins, and gums. A number of such forest products are used locally, while a few enter into the foreign commerce of the Islands. The present bulletin aims to present a somewhat popular account of these various products.

A short account of agricultural, oil-yielding plants has been included for the sake of completeness. This has seemed the more advisable as there are only a few of them. The most important oil-producing plants, which can be regarded as strictly agricultural and never wild, are the coconut palm and peanut. There are in the Philippines a number of cultivated medicinal plants which contain oils. They are, however, for the most part unimportant, and oil is not extracted from them in the Archipelago.

Some of the resinous products and seed oils from Philippine forests are used extensively in the preparation of paints and varnishes, while others are employed for medicinal purposes, illumination, the manufacture of soaps, etc. A number of the resins, which occur most abundantly, are of comparatively little value at the present time, but some of these would seem to have promising possibilities.

A few of the Philippine essential oils (the odoriferous, volatile oils obtained from vegetable sources) are used commercially in the preparation of perfumes; and others would be valuable commercially, if this industry were properly developed. *Acacia farnesiana* (aroma) is a very common species in grasslands and open places in the Philippines. In France this shrub is grown extensively for the perfume obtained from its flowers, known as cassie flowers. There is no record of such a utilization in the Philippines.

The chief difficulty encountered in the collection of products from Philippine forest trees is that the forests usually contain a large number of species, so that a given species, although of wide distribution, may occur only in small numbers in a limited area. Many of the Philippine oil-producing plants grow well under cultivation, and the greatest development of oil industries from such plants will be dependent on their being grown in plantations by private individuals or in reforestation projects. A beginning has already been made in this direction, and in the case of *Canangium odoratum* (ilang-ilang) the oil is distilled largely from flowers grown under cultivation. *Aleurites moluccana,* the source of lumbang oil, is fairly common in some regions, and the oil, which is extracted commercially, is largely from wild trees. This species and also *Aleurites trisperma,* the source of bagilumbang oil, grow rapidly in plantations, and the trees fruit in a few years. These species are very promising for plantation and reforestation projects, and great numbers have already been planted. It can, therefore, be safely predicted that the future supply of lumbang and bagilumbang oils will be mostly from planted trees. As these oils are valuable, there are bright prospects for the development of a considerable industry in the handling of them. Several other oil-producing species which have been tried in limited quantities in plantations give promise of doing well. Among them may be mentioned *Pongamia pinnata, Sterculia foetida, Terminalia catappa,* and *Sindora supa. Canarium luzonicum,* the source of Manila elemi, also apparently does well in plantations. It would thus seem that the Manila elemi industry can best be developed from planted trees. This is probably likewise true of *Canarium villosum* and *Agathis alba,* although the latter species occurs in considerable abundance.

While most of the oil plants and some of the resinous ones grow for the most part as scattered individuals, this is not true of all the resin-producing trees. *Pinus insularis* grows in pure stands of considerable extent in the mountain regions of central Luzon, and *Pinus merkusii* in Mindoro. Most of the species of the family Dipterocarpaceae are large and dominant trees and grow in such numbers that immense quantities of resin could be produced. Unfortunately there is comparatively little market for these resins, although balau, from *Dipterocarpus vernicifluus, D. grandiflorus,* and other species of *Dipterocarpus,* and *Anisoptera thurifera,* appears to be very promising as a source of varnish resin and could be obtained in very large quantities. According to Foxworthy,* the species of *Dipterocarpus* make up

---

* Foxworthy, F. W., Philippine Dipterocarpaceae, II. Philippine Journal of Science, Section C, Volume 13 (1918), page 163.

20 per cent of the volume of the commercial forests of the Philippines.

Among cultivated species there are several which seem to offer promising prospects for the establishment of considerable industries. *Elaeis guineensis* (oil palm), which is used in the Philippines only for ornamental purposes, grows very well and is apparently not attacked by insects or fungi. In Africa this plant is grown very extensively for the oil derived from the seeds. Large plantations are also being started in Sumatra. Peanuts are raised in considerable quantities, but very little oil is extracted. In many countries, peanut oil is a commercial product of great importance. Sesame, which is grown in India and other countries on a huge scale for the production of sesame oil, grows well in the Philippines, but is cultivated only to a limited extent, and the oil is extracted merely for local purposes. Palm, peanut, and sesame oils are used extensively for edible purposes and for the manufacture of soap. *Achras sapota* (chico) is cultivated in the Philippines for its edible fruit. This species is grown extensively in Mexico for the production of gum chicle, the principal material employed in the manufacture of chewing-gum.

From the above discussion of oils, resins, and gums, it will be seen that there are promising prospects for the development of industries which already exist and for the establishment of a number of new ones.

RESINS

Resins and gums are products obtained from the exudations of plants. The products may exude spontaneously, but are more often secured by making incisions in the bark or trunk. It is somewhat difficult to draw a sharp distinction between gums and resins, as there are a number of plant exudations known as oleoresins, balsams and gum resins which have properties intermediate between those of true gums and resins. In general, plant products of this nature contain resins, gums, volatile oils, and aromatic acids. Allen * gives a very satisfactory discussion of resins and the methods used in analyzing them.

Resins are solid or semi-solid and are usually insoluble in water, but soluble in alcohol, ether, and volatile oils. They are formed usually by the spontaneous evaporation of resinous juices which exude naturally from the trunks of trees or when the trunks are cut. Frequently resins may be extracted from various parts of plants by solvents such as alcohol and ether. They are also found as minerals (mineral resin) which are, no doubt, products of extinct vegetation. Resins from different sources frequently show great differences in their chemical composition and properties. Commercially, Manila copal, which is used in making varnishes, is the most important Philippine resin.

Oleoresins are the plant exudations consisting of resins dissolved in volatile essential oils. Manila elemi, employed in varnish making, and turpentine are examples of this class of substances occurring in the Philippines.

Gum resins are plant exudations, like gamboge, which consist of a mixture of resin and gum. Gamboge of an inferior quality' can be obtained in the Philippines from *Garcinia venulosa* and probably from other species of *Garcinia*.

Certain of the dipterocarp resins can be collected in large quantities and appear to offer commercial possibilities as materials for the manufacture of varnishes.

Family PINACEAE
Genus AGATHIS

AGATHIS ALBA (Lam.) Foxw. (Figs. 2–4). ALMÁCIGA.

Local names: *Adiáñgau* (Camarines); *alinsagó* (Benguet); *almáciga* (Mindoro, Lepanto, Bataan, Tayabas, Benguet, Zambales, Palawan, Cama-

---

* Allen, Commercial organic analysis, Volume 4 (1911), page 1.

16

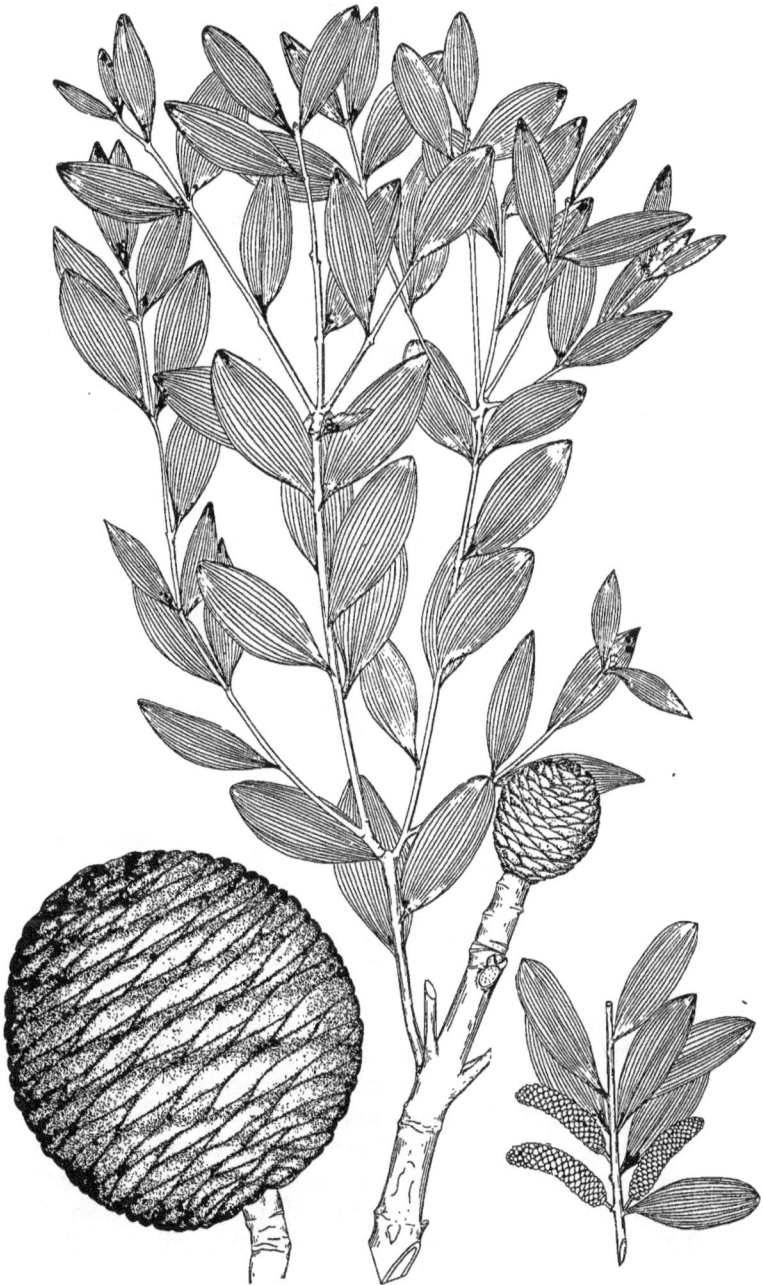

FIGURE 2. AGATHIS ALBA (ALMÁCIGA), THE SOURCE OF MANILA COPAL. $\times\frac{1}{2}$.

rines, Negros); *almaciga babae* (Bataan); *aniñgá* (Isabela); *aniñgát* (Calayan Island); *ánteng* (Nueva Ecija); *bagtík, baltík* (Palawan); *biáyo* (Bisaya); *bidiáñgan* (Negros Occidental); *bunsóg* (Benguet); *dadiáñgau* (Sorsogon, Polillo, Tayabas, Negros); *dadúñgoi* (Albay, Sorsogon); *galagála* (Bataan, Palawan); *ladiáñgau* (Camarines, Sorsogon, Tayabas); *makáu* (Misamis); *pino* (Samar); *sálong* (Cagayan, Negros); *títau* (Abra); *úli* (Zambales).

ALMACIGA OR MANILA COPAL

The chief value of *Agathis alba* is in the resin (almaciga or Manila copal) which it yields. Locally this is employed as incense in religious ceremonies, for torches, starting fires, caulking boats, as a smudge for mosquitoes, etc. It is exported in considerable quantities, and used chiefly in the manufacture of high-grade varnish, but also in other processes, as in making patent leather and sealing wax. Almaciga is suitable, according to Richmond,[*] for the manufacture of cheap soaps and paper size. Aqueous solutions of the alkaline resinates are precipitated by solutions of all other metallic salts, e. g., aluminum sulphate, in the form of an insoluble resinate, which could be used in paper manufacturing to render the paper non-bibulous. The exports of almaciga from the Philippines from 1914 to 1918 are given in Table 1.

TABLE 1.—*Amount and value of Manila copal exported from the Philippines from 1914 to 1918.*

Year.	Amount.	Value.
	Kilograms.	*Pesos.*
1914	1,112,787	225,078
1915	1,304,975	206,446
1916	1,143,938	211,593
1917	593,560	188,940
1918	507,116	138,821

Agathis alba belongs to the pine family and to the same genus as the "kauri pine" (*Agathis robusta*) of New Zealand. The latter yields a resin very similar to almaciga and one which has long been important in the industries.

Manila copal is a member of the class of substances known as copals. These substances are obtained as resinous exudations from various trees or as fossil (mineral) resin and are used principally for manufacturing varnishes. According to Hyde:[†]

---

[*] Richmond, G. F., Manila copal. Philippine Journal of Science, Section A, Volume 5 (1910), pages 177 to 201.

[†] Hyde, F. S., Solvents, oils, gums, waxes and allied substances (1913), page 35.

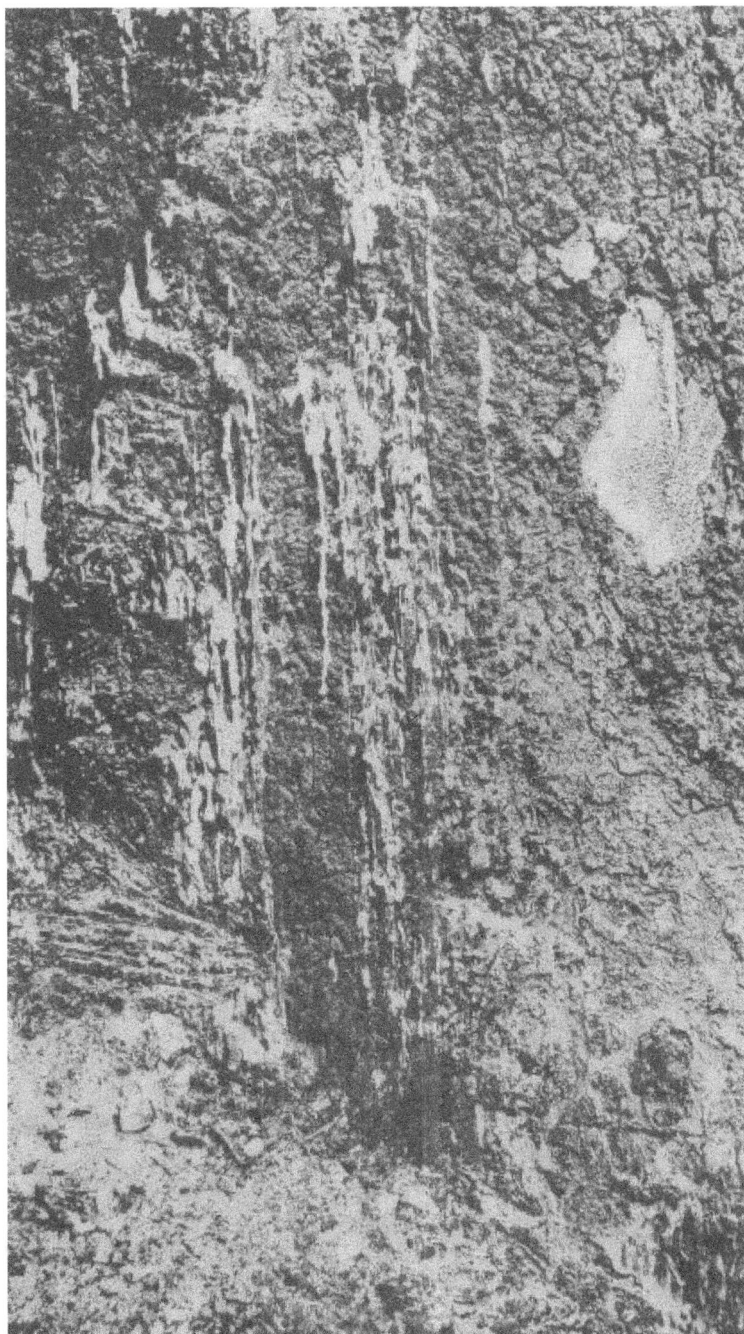

FIGURE 3. TRUNK OF AGATHIS ALBA (ALMÁCIGA), WITH SCARS FROM WHICH
MANILA COPAL IS EXUDING.

True copals are hard, lustrous, yellow, brown, or nearly white, and more or less insoluble in the usual solvents, but are rendered soluble by melting before making into varnish.

The copals are resins which contain those very permanent substances known as resenes.

Bottler and Sabin * state that:

* * * they contain, moreover, ethereal oils, which are driven off by melting or distillation, a bitter principle, and coloring-matter. Zanzibar and Cameroon copals consist mainly of resin acids and resenes; * * * Manila is composed mostly of resin acids; but it contains more resene (12 per cent) than does Zanzibar (6 per cent). * * *

Bottler and Sabin † further say:

For making spirit copal varnishes only such copals can be used as will readily dissolve to a clear solution, free from slimy or stringy qualities. Manila and Borneo copals are used, the soft Angola and the newer Sierra Leone.

These varnishes may be made by such formulas as the following:

		Parts.
(a)	Manila copal	16
	Venice turpentine	4 to 5
	Alcohol (95 per cent)	30

The resin of *Agathis alba* is found in the bark, and oozes out whenever the latter is cut (surface resin). Occasionally lumps of resin are found in the forks of branches, and large masses, the so-called fossil (mineral) resins, are found in the ground. These deposits are located by sounding the ground with sharp-pointed sticks. Such resin is often discovered in places where large trees have formerly stood, but which have long since died and decayed, leaving large masses of resin in the ground.

According to Richmond,‡ more than 50 per cent of the Manila copal exported from the Philippines is collected in the Davao district of Mindanao, and probably 90 per cent of the resin produced in that region is obtained by blazing living trees. The best results are secured by removing, from different sides of trees, strips of bark about one meter in length and 20 to 30 centimeters wide, thus providing clean surfaces on which the resin is deposited as it oozes from the cut end of the bark. The resin is also obtained by means of a wedge-shaped incision in the tree trunk. This method however does not provide a clean

---

* Bottler, M. and Sabin, A. H., German and American varnish making (1912), page 13.

† Bottler, M. and Sabin, A. H., German and American varnish making (1912), page 131.

‡ Richmond, G. F., Manila copal. Philippine Journal of Science, Section A, Volume 5 (1910), pages 177 to 201.

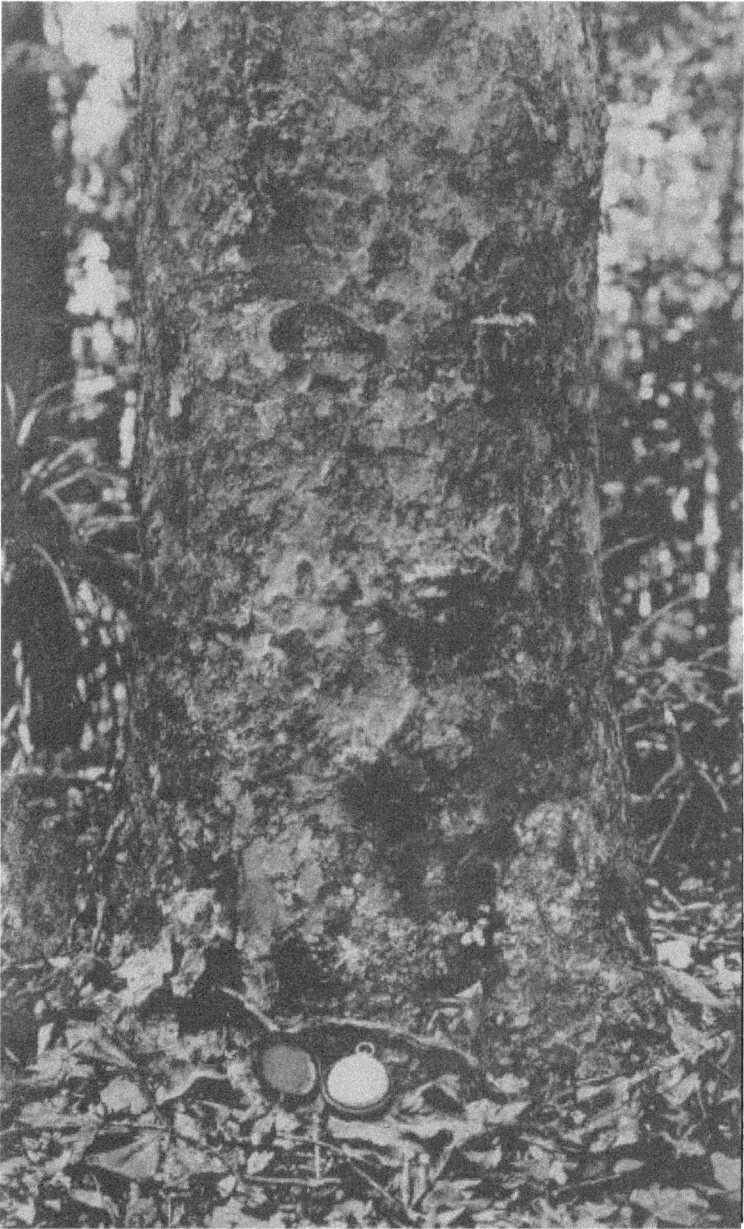

FIGURE 4. TRUNK OF AGATHIS ALBA (ALMÁCIGA), THE SOURCE OF MANILA COPAL.

surface, and the resulting resin is generally mixed with chips of bark.

When the resin first exudes from the tree, it appears as almost colorless tears, the outer surfaces of which soon harden. As exudation continues, the fresh resin instead of flowing out over the first portion produced appears to force the latter outward by being deposited beneath it. The outer surfaces are thus always hard and friable and the inner portion hardens very slowly. About two weeks are required to produce solid pieces of marketable size.

The Manila copal which is exported from the Philippines directly to the United States is cleaned, sorted, and graded in Manila. Particular attention is paid to cleanliness, color, and size. Manila copal is sometimes adulterated with other resins, particularly dipterocarp resins; the latter, however, are very readily distinguished from Manila copal. As the resin is collected largely by non-Christian tribes, the sorters in Manila frequently encounter considerable admixtures of other resins, and as the consumers have to depend largely on Philippine sorters, it is not surprising that the securing of a uniform quality of resin is a matter of some difficulty.

ANALYSIS OF MANILA COPAL

Almaciga has been the subject of a number of investigations by the Bureau of Science.*

Richmond examined recent surface and fossil (mineral) resin to ascertain the probable composition and character of these substances. The acid value was determined by dissolving approximately one gram of powdered resin in 50 cubic centimeters of absolute alcohol and titrating with a half-normal solution of alcoholic potassium hydroxide, using phenolphthalein as an indicator. A gram of surface resin required approximately 128 milligrams of potash for neutralization, while a gram of mineral resin required about 110.

The saponification value was determined in the following manner:—About one gram of resin was dissolved in 50 cubic centimeters of absolute alcohol. Twenty-five cubic centimeters

* Foxworthy, F. W., The almaciga tree: *Agathis alba* (Lam.), Philippine Journal of Science, Section A, Volume 5 (1910), pages 173 to 175.

Richmond, G. F., Manila copal. Philippine Journal of Science, Section A, Volume 5 (1910), pages 177 to 201.

Brooks, B. T., The destructive distillation of Manila copal. Philippine Journal of Science, Section A, Volume 5 (1910), pages 203 to 217.

Brooks, B. T., The oxidation of Manila copal by the air. Philippine Journal of Science, Section A, Volume 5 (1910), pages 219 to 227.

of half-normal alcoholic potash were then added and the mixture heated on a steam bath (refluxed) for an hour. The excess of potassium hydroxide was titrated with a half-normal alcoholic solution of hydrogen chloride. A gram of surface resin required approximately 177 milligrams of potassium hydroxide for neutralization, while a gram of fossil resin took about 150 milligrams. The acid and saponification values of various samples of resin were determined. The results showed that darker specimens of resin gave higher acid and saponification values than did lighter-colored ones.

Samples of surface resin were distilled with steam, but only traces of volatile oil were obtained. Fossil resin which was finely pulverized yielded a larger proportion of volatile oil. When steam-distilled in the presence of an alkali, 500 grams of surface resin gave 6.5 grams of oil, while an equal quantity of fossil resin gave 40 grams of oil. The oil obtained by steam distillation when dried over solid potassium hydroxide had a pale-lemon color and pleasant odor. This was fractionally distilled. The main fraction boiled between 155° and 165°. By treating with hydrochloric acid gas this fraction was converted into a hydrochloride which crystallized from alcohol and melted at 124°. This substance was identified as pinene hydrochloride.

A method of analysis devised by Richmond showed that one hundred parts of crude resin gave the following results:

	Parts.
Insoluble in absolute alcohol	.5
Soluble in alcoholic potash	40.0
Insoluble in alcoholic potash	41.5
Neutral oil soluble in alcohol and volatile with steam..	6.0
Neutral resin partially soluble in alcohol and non-volatile with steam	10.0
Water, etc., undetermined	2.0

These results confirm the conclusion of Tschirch that Manila copal consists mainly of amorphous free resin acids, and contains a neutral resin indifferent to alkalies, and a volatile oil. Richmond extracted the resin acids from Manila copal by using a modification of Tschirch's method. An ether extract of Manila copal was treated with 5 per cent ammonium carbonate solution for several days, after which the mixture was acidified. The resin acids were precipitated as an amorphous powder. When this precipitate was dissolved in dilute alcohol and crystallized, white crystals melting at 186° were obtained. Analysis showed that these crystals had the molecular formula $C_{10}H_{15}O_2$ and that the resin acid was monobasic.

MANILA COPAL AS AN INGREDIENT OF VARNISHES.

As previously stated, Manila copal is used principally as an ingredient of varnishes. Spirit varnishes are solutions of resin in a volatile solvent such as turpentine, benzene, alcohol or some other solvent. Plain oil varnishes consist of only linseed oil or some other drying oil. The oleoresinous varnishes contain all the ingredients of both spirit and plain oil varnishes, and have properties common to both. The manufacture of oleoresinous varnishes consists essentially in mixing resin, turpentine, and a drying oil, such as linseed oil, in the proper proportions. Usually resins do not dissolve readily in drying oils unless the mixture is heated somewhat, and even then the resin frequently separates upon cooling. It is therefore customary to heat both the oil and resin before and after mixing. Richmond showed that although Manila copal loses weight when heated, the melted resin differs from the raw resin only in the amount and nature of unsaponifiable matter, that is, in the free amorphous acids. He concluded that the resin which enters into varnish manufacture consists essentially of free acids of the same composition as the free acids in the original copal, and that there is no particular reason for heating the resin to a high temperature either before or after mixing. He found that oleic, palmitic, and linolic acids dissolve the resin acids of Manila copal at moderate temperature.

A quantity of the mixed fatty acids of linseed oil was prepared and added in varying proportions to raw linseed oil, depending upon the quantity of unmelted resin it was desired to dissolve, and it was found that raw or boiled linseed oil, containing the free, mixed, fatty acids of linseed oil in the proportions of 10 to 30 per cent calculated as oleïc acid, formed homogeneous solutions with raw or fused Manila copal when the latter is added in the proportion of 10 to 30 gallon varnishes and heated for a time at a maximum of 200°. When the turpentine was added before the oil, the boiling point of turpentine, 155° to 165°, was sufficiently high to effect complete solution with the exception of such foreign matter as may be present in the resin. The subsequent addition of turpentine to the oil and resin did not produce any cloudiness.

Varnish prepared as described above was used for varnishing native hardwood. The varnish film remained a year without showing any appreciable loss of luster.

Richmond concluded that:

The changes which take place during the cooking of varnish are largely changes in the oil rather than the resin, i. e., it is possible so to treat linseed oil, either by boiling or by adding to it linseed-oil acids previous to its addition to the fused resin, that it will form a clear, homogeneous mixture with the latter which will remain so upon cooling, without subsequent heating to temperatures greater than 150° to 200°.

Richmond also prepared an oleoresinous varnish entirely from Philippine raw materials, consisting of lumbang oil, Manila copal, and turpentine. The lumbang was used in place of linseed as a drying oil. The turpentine was obtained by distilling the resin of the Benguet pine. Red narra wood, which had received two coats of this varnish, remained exposed for over a year without any appreciable loss of luster.

DISTILLATION OF MANILA COPAL

Brooks * carried out a number of experiments on the distillation of Manila copal. His results verified the observations of other experimenters that the distillation takes place in two stages. The first stage is characterized by considerable frothing. As the temperature rises slowly to about 330° the mass becomes fluid and boils gently. The loss in weight at this stage is about 14 per cent of the original sample. At about 340° the resin oil distils over in large quantities. The weight of oil obtained from 1,500 grams of resin was 94 grams. The fraction boiling between 150° and 178° gave 24 grams of oil, and contained limonene, pinene, terpineol, iso-borneol and β-pinene.

TABLE 2.—*Substances given off by Manila copal during the first stage of the decomposition, up to 330°.*

Substances.	Per cent.
Carbon dioxide	3.2
Water	2.4
Formic acid and acetic acid .... each....	0.5
Formaldehyde, acetyl formaldehyde, furfuraldehyde, methyl alcohol, and acetone, approximately	0.2
Gaseous hydrocarbons	0.2
Pinene, limonene, dipentene, β-pinene, and camphene, variable	1.5–11.2
Resin oil, variable, usually from	3.0–6.0

Brooks also analyzed the gases given off during the first stage of the distillation of Manila copal and ascertained the quantity of carbon dioxide, unsaturated hydrocarbons, and saturated hydrocarbons. The principal products obtained by distilling Manila copal up to a temperature of 330° are given in Table 2. The solubility of Manila copal in various solvents was determined, with the results given in Table 3. These results are, however, only approximate, as different pieces vary somewhat in solubility.

---

* Brooks, B. T., Destructive distillation of Manila copal. Philippine Journal of Science, Section A, volume 5 (1910), page 203.

TABLE 3.—*Per cent of substance dissolved from 10 grams of resin by 100 cubic centimeters of solvent.*

Solvent.	Per cent.	Temperature used to expel solvent.
		°C
Ethyl alcohol	95	130
Amyl alcohol	97	150-155
Ether	75	120
Ligroin	32	130
Benzene	50	135-140
Turpentine	46	170-175

OXIDATION OF MANILA COPAL

The absorption of oxygen from the air appears to be a property common to all complex resin acids. Brooks * investigated the oxidation of Manila copal by air and summarized his results as follows:

1. Manila copal rapidly absorbs oxygen from the air. The oxidation is accompanied by the formation of organic peroxides, an increase in the Koettstorfer number, and evolution of small quantities of carbon dioxide, formaldehyde, formic acid, and hydrogen peroxide.

2. The resin acids of Manila copal, when separated from the terpenes occurring in the natural resin, undergo oxidation by the air.

3. The evolution of carbon dioxide from Manila copal and colophony is probably due to the formation of organic peroxides and their subsequent decomposition.

4. The increase in the Koettstorfer number obtained by prolonged digestion with alcoholic potassium hydroxide is not due to oxidation during the course of the experiment, but is probably caused, at least in part, by the breaking down of lactones and organic peroxides. Samples which have been exposed to the air give up carbon dioxide and formic acid to the alkaline solution in the Koettstorfer determination and cause the recovered resin to show lower Koettstorfer numbers than the initial values.

5. Formaldehyde has heretofore not been noted among the products of the oxidation of organic substances by the air. I have found it among the products of the atmospheric oxidation of Manila copal.

6. The oxidation of Manila copal by the air is accelerated by sunlight.

Ingle † examined Manila copal to ascertain the effect of exposing it to the air. The material was finely ground and ex-

* Brooks, B. T., Oxidation of Manila copal by the air. Philippine Journal of Science, Section A, Volume 5 (1910), page 219.

† Ingle, H., Some notes on gum resins. Journal of the Society of Chemical Industry, Volume 31 (1912), page 272.

posed to light and air. At intervals of 78 days, 13 months, and 2 years, the copal was weighed and the acid and iodine values determined. His results showed that the acid value was practically unchanged while the iodine value decreased. He also determined the solubility of Manila copal in various solvents, and suggested a method for estimating Manila copal in the presence of other resins. He believed that Manila copal, which is cheaper than kauri resin, could be used in place of the latter in certain dental-mould preparations.

DESCRIPTION AND DISTRIBUTION OF AGATHIS ALBA

Agathis alba is a large tree reaching a height of 50 to 60 meters and a diameter, at breast height, of more than 2 meters; and with a clear length of trunk of 30 meters or more. The bark is 10 to 15 millimeters in thickness, brittle, and light greenish to brownish gray in color. It is shed in scroll-shaped patterns and is thickly set with corky pustules. The inner bark is brown, streaked with red and grading into a cream color near the sapwood. The leaves are simple, opposite or nearly so, leathery in texture, 3 to 9.5 centimeters long, and 1 to 2.5 centimeters wide.

The wood is moderately hard, flexible, and tough, though not resilient. The heartwood is pale yellow, sometimes with a faint pinkish or brownish tinge, generally turning to an even, very pale brown in drying.

This species was first described at length by Rumphius, who called it *Dammara alba*, which is the Latin form of the Malay common name, dammár putí. The same name was used by Lamarck in 1786, but the genus has since come to be known as *Agathis*, a name which is retained in the Vienna Code.

Agathis alba is found growing in considerable numbers in forests at altitudes of from 200 to 2,000 meters, but in the Philippines it usually attains its best development on well-drained slopes at from 600 to 1,500 meters elevation. The tree is very common in the Philippines and exists on mountain slopes throughout the Archipelago. It has been reported from the following regions: Cagayan, Isabela, Lepanto, Benguet, Abra, Zambales, Nueva Ecija, Bataan, Rizal, Tayabas, Polillo, Mindoro, Camarines, Albay, Sorsogon, Calayan Island, Sibuyan, Negros, Samar, Palawan, Misamis, Davao, and Zamboanga. *Agathis alba* also occurs in Cochin China, the Malay Peninsula, Sumatra, Java, Celebes, the Moluccas, and Borneo.

Genus PINUS

PINUS INSULARIS Endl.   (Figs. 5–7).   SÁLENG * or BENGUET PINE.

Local names: *Alál* (Zambales); *balibo, boobóo, bulbúl, ol-ól, sáung* (Benguet); *parua* (Iloko); *sáleng* (Bontoc, Lepanto, Abra, Nueva Ecija, Ilocos Norte and Sur).

TURPENTINE

Two species of pines are natives of the Philippines, one of which, *Pinus insularis*, was used in Spanish times as a commercial source of turpentine. Richmond † says that turpentine collected from this tree has an appearance and consistency somewhat like that of crystallized honey and possesses a pleasant odor; while Brooks ‡, after an investigation, states that it is practically identical with that produced in America. Brooks measured the flow from a number of trees. Concerning the results he writes §:

On March 13, fourteen trees situated in the forest adjoining the claim of the Headwaters Mining Company were boxed. The trees were selected at random and included several trees of the variety known to lumbermen and turpentine collectors as "scrub pine." Six hours later thirteen of the trees showed an abundant flow of resin, while one was hard and did not flow. The collected resin weighed 1,761.5 grams.

On March 14, thirty trees were boxed in another locality about 2 miles distant from Baguio. They were selected with the idea of including both healthy and unhealthy looking trees and some which had been damaged by ground fires. On the following day these trees were again visited and all but three, which were hard and did not flow, were still running slowly. The collected resin weighed 4,400 grams.

Method of boxing.—The boxes were cut about 30 to 40 centimeters wide, 12 to 18 centimeters deep, and 6 to 8 centimeters from front to back, varying with the size of the trees. They were made by inexperienced laborers and were so badly split and bruised that much of the fresh resin was lost, hence the yields obtained do not accurately represent the total flow of resin.

One of the best flowing trees had a diameter of about 85 centimeters and produced 857 grams of resin in thirty-two hours, although a portion was lost by overflowing the box.

----

* The words *sálong, sáleng, sáhing* and *sáing, sáong* or *sáung*, which occur so constantly as local names of trees of the Pine, Pili, and Lauan families (Pinaceae, Burseraceae, and Dipterocarpaceae), are all various dialectic forms of one word having the general meaning of "resin."

† Richmond, G. F., Philippine turpentine. Philippine Journal of Science, Section A, Volume 4 (1909), pages 231 to 232.

‡ Brooks, B. T., The oleoresin of Pinus insularis Endl. Philippine Journal of Science, Section A, Volume 5 (1910), pages 229 to 231.

§ Richmond, G. F., Philippine turpentine. Philippine Journal of Science, Section A, Volume 4 (1909), page 231.

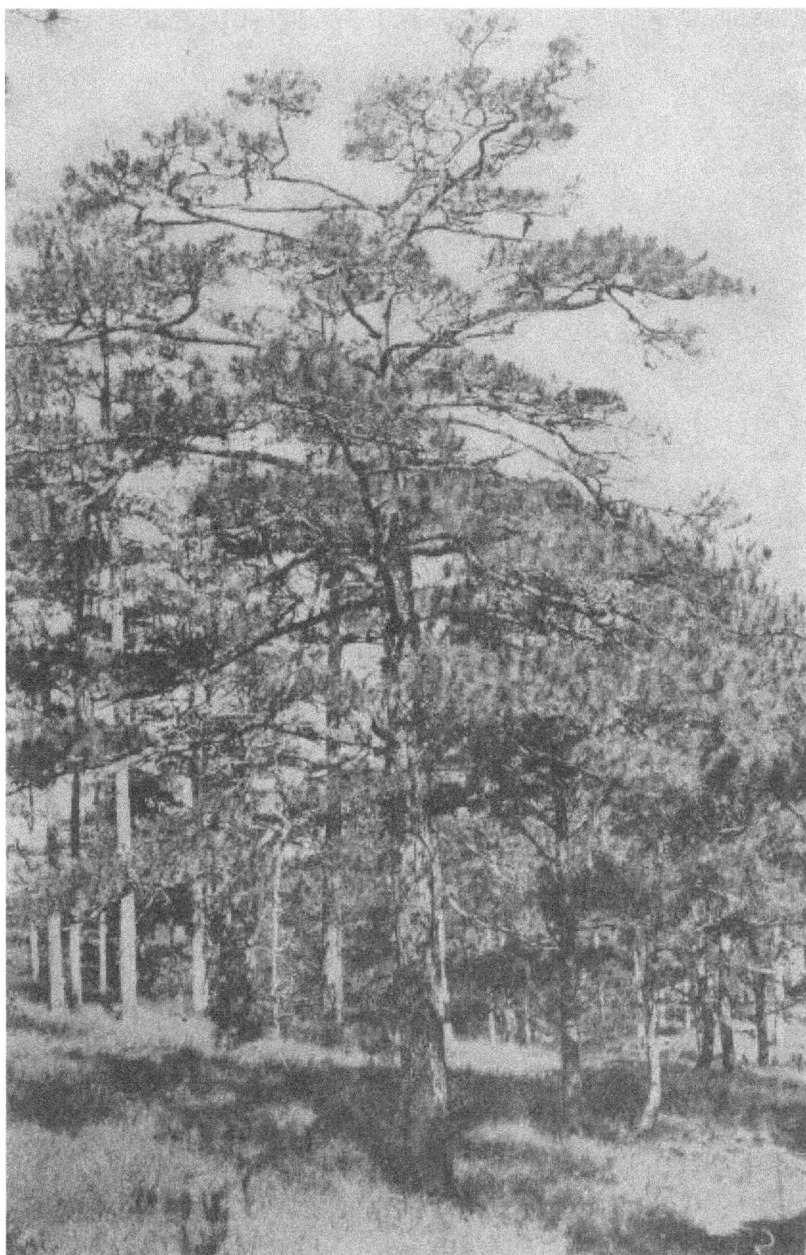

FIGURE 5. FOREST OF PINUS INSULARIS (BENGUET PINE) IN BENGUET MOUNTAINS.

These samples being taken during the dry season probably represent a smaller yield than would be obtained during the rainy season when the trees have more life and the loss by evaporation is less.

The cup and gutter system of collection would also give large yields by minimizing the loss.

Richmond * investigated the turpentine obtained from *Pinus insularis* and found that exhaustive distillation of the resin gave 412.2 grams (23.4 per cent) of oil of turpentine which was water-white in color, and after drying over calcium chloride gave the following results: Specific gravity, $\frac{30°}{30°}=0.8593$; refractive index, $N\frac{30°}{D}=1.4656$; optical rotation, $A\frac{30°}{D}=+26.5$. Ninety-six per cent distilled between 154° and 165.5°.

The residue from the steam distillation amounted to 76.6 per cent of the original resin and was freed from approximately 15 grams of foreign material by hot filtration. It consisted of pine colophony of a clear, pale-amber color.

Brooks † collected samples of the oleoresin from different trees and steam-distilled them, after which he determined the optical rotations. The values he obtained at 30° (+13.15° to +27.48°) were not very uniform, but the differences were not as large as those noted by Herty in the case of American turpentine.

The constants and chemical properties of the turpentine obtained from *Pinus insularis* indicate that the oil consists principally of pinene. Several derivatives of pinene, such as pinene nitrosyl chloride, were prepared from the turpentine. Brooks concluded that the turpentine and colophony from *Pinus insularis* are practically identical with those produced in America.

Pinus insularis reaches a height of 40 meters and a diameter of 140 centimeters. The bole is straight and clear, the crown narrow, with the lateral branches weakly developed. The bark is 10 to 25 millimeters in thickness, yellow or reddish brown in color, and broken in sections by vertical and horizontal cracks. The leaves are grouped in bunches of three, or sometimes two, and are 8 to·30 centimeters in length. The wood is moderately hard and heavy, resembling the yellow pine of the United States.

* Richmond, G. F., Philippine turpentine. Philippine Journal of Science, Section A, Volume 4 (1909), page 231.

† Brooks, B. T., The oleoresin of Pinus insularis Endl. Philippine Journal of Science, Section A, Volume 5 (1910), page 229.

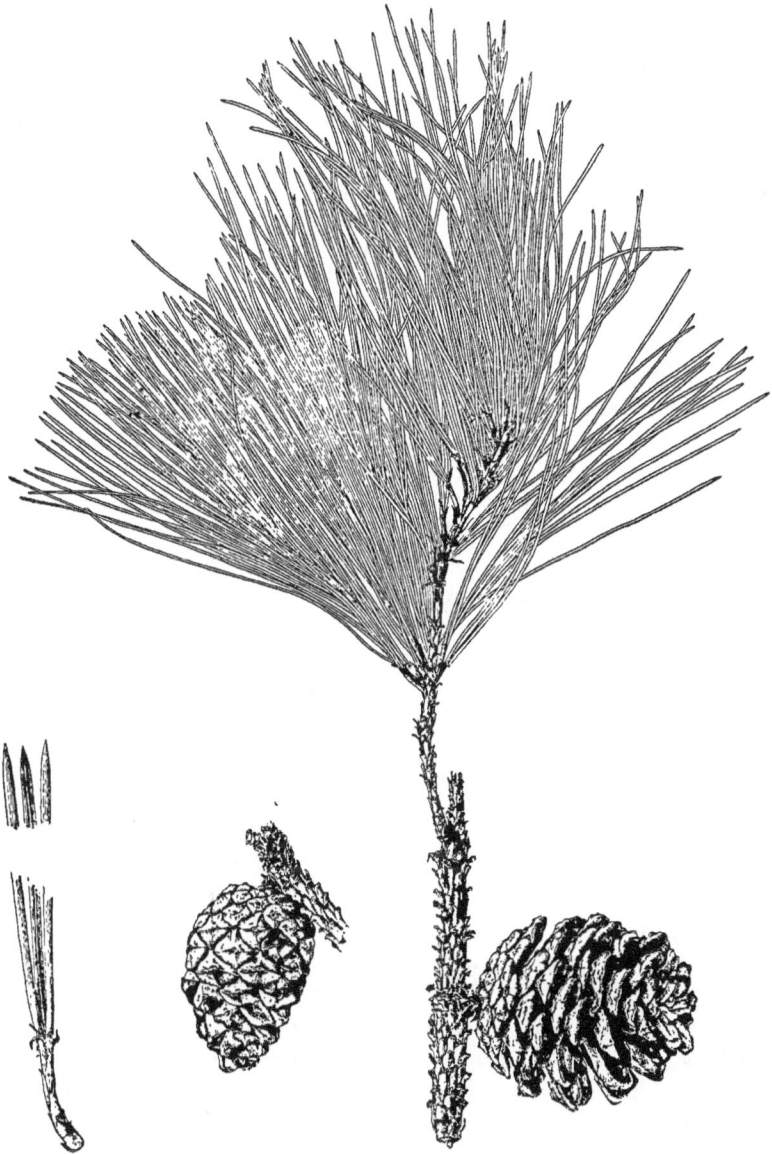

JVitan deL

FIGURE 6. PINUS INSULARIS (BENGUET PINE), A SOURCE OF TURPENTINE.

The sapwood is white; the heartwood white and reddish brown with alternate light and dark rings, and very resinous. It is used locally for house construction, mining props, etc.

This species is found in the highlands of central and northern Luzon at altitudes varying from 500 to 2,500 meters, but is best developed at altitudes ranging from 900 to 1,500 meters. The stands vary in density from those composed of scattered individuals to nearly closed patches. The ground in a pine area is usually covered with grass. In the ravines, broad-leaved trees occur and there is considerable evidence to show that nearly the whole area now occupied by the pines was formerly covered by broad-leaved trees, the pines being confined to steeper and dryer situations, where the other trees did not flourish. Through the activities of man in past centuries, the broad-leaved trees have been cleared off, and repeated fires have prevented their reproduction. The result of successive fires is usually to leave the lands in possession of grasses. The pines are less susceptible to fire than are the broad-leaved trees and consequently the former occur over wide areas. If fires were kept out, the pine, in the absence of competition with the broad-leaved trees, would quickly occupy the entire area, as its reproduction is abundant and rapid. The pines would then gradually be replaced by broad-leaved trees, as these will seed under the pines and cast such a dense shade as to prevent the growth of pine seedlings.

Measurements show a volume of 74 cubic meters per hectare (equivalent to about 7,400 board feet per acre) of pine trees which have a diameter of 25 or more centimeters.

PINUS MERKUSII Jungh. (Fig. 8).   TAPÚLAU or MINDORO PINE.
Local names: *Agú-u* (Mindoro); *salit, tapúlau* (Zambales).

TURPENTINE

This species has not been investigated chemically, but its products are probably similar to those of *Pinus insularis*. The wood is apparently identical with the latter species, but seems on the average to be even more resinous.

Pinus merkusii is a tree reaching a diameter of about 90 centimeters. The chief difference between this species and *Pinus insularis* is that the needles occur in groups of two rather than three.

This species is found in Zambales and northwestern Mindoro, occurring in the latter region in pure stands. In Zambales, both *Pinus merkusii* and *Pinus insularis* aré found at altitudes of only one or two hundred meters.

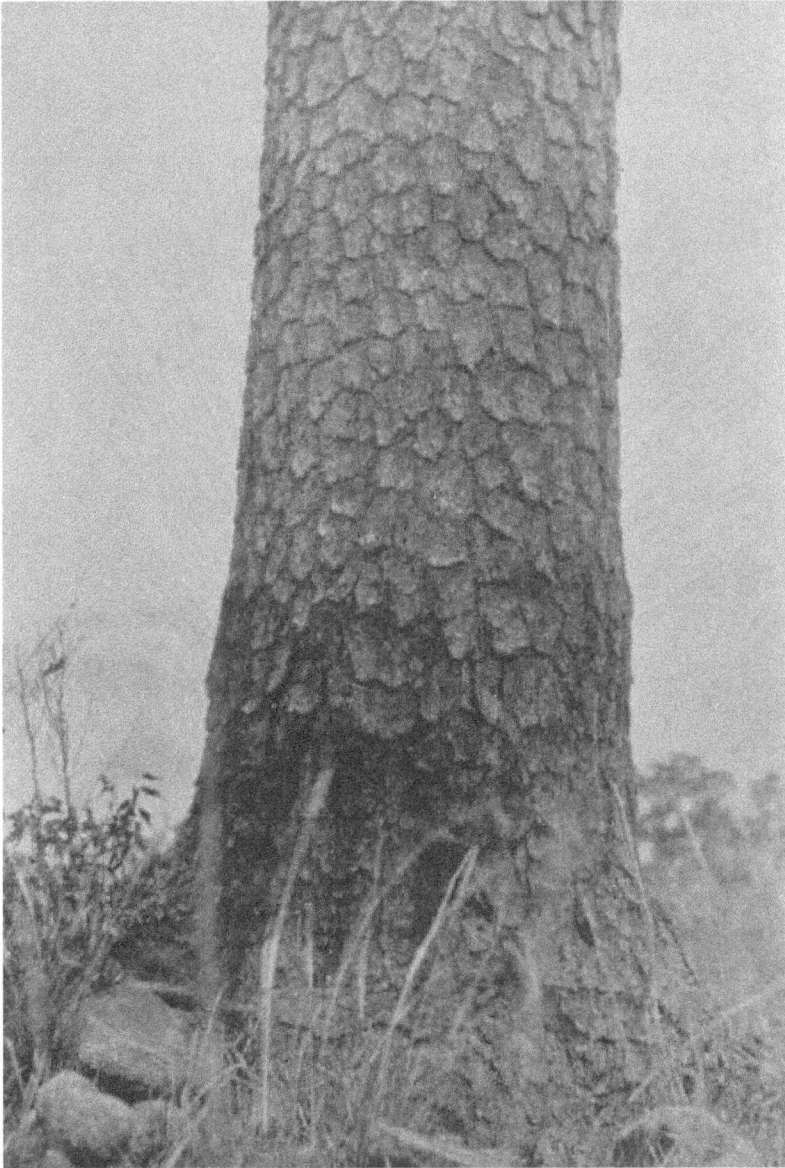

FIGURE 7. TRUNK OF PINUS INSULARIS (BENGUET PINE).

168837——3

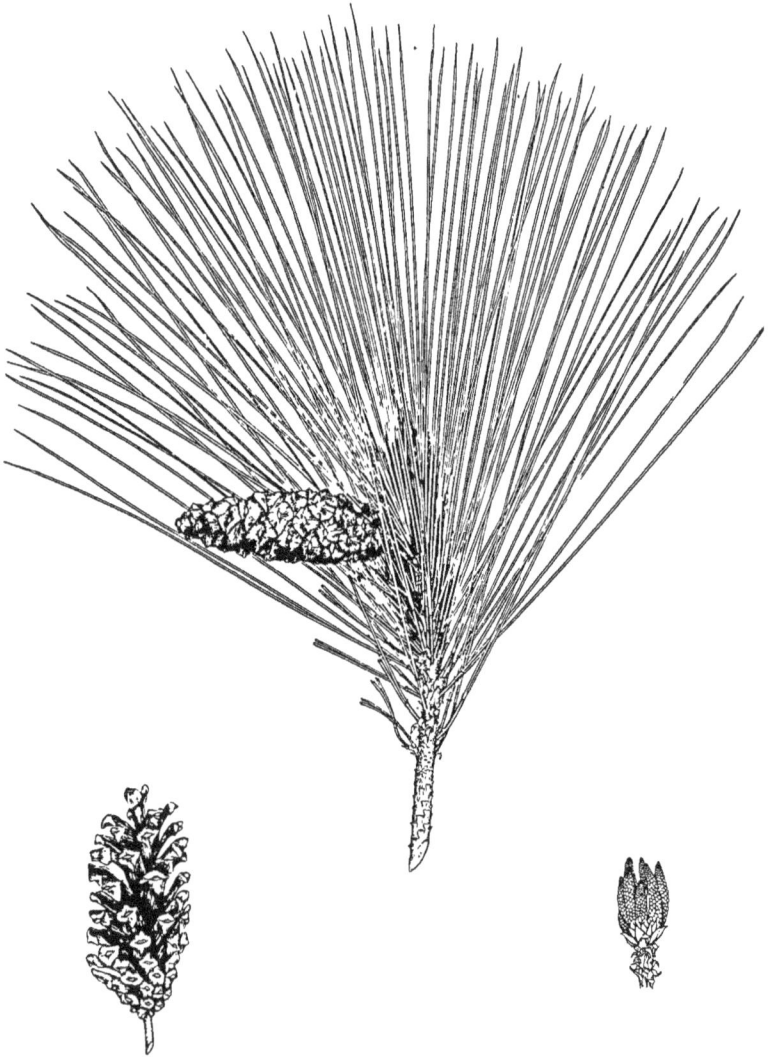

FIGURE 8. PINUS MERKUSII (MINDORO PINE), A SOURCE OF TURPENTINE. ×⅓.

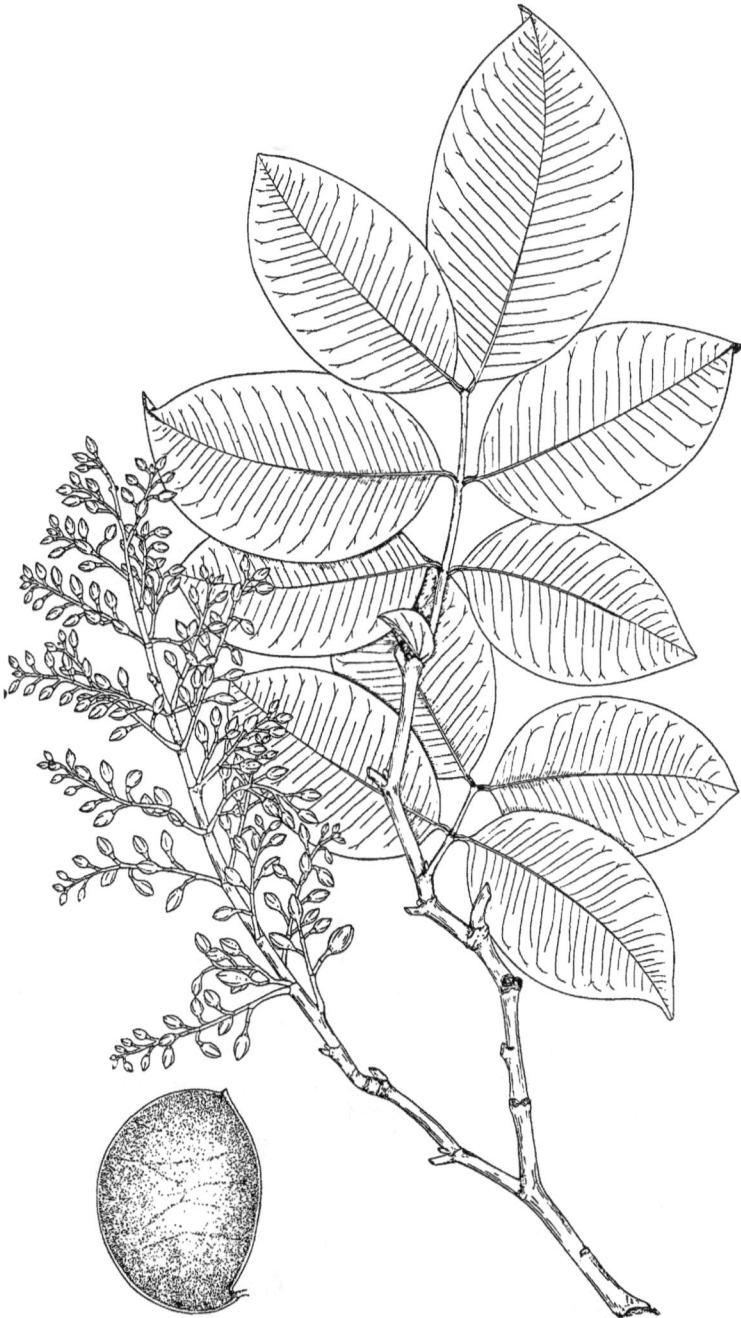

FIGURE 9. SINDORA INERMIS (KAYU-GÁLU), THE SOURCE OF KAYU-GÁLU OIL. ×½.

FAMILY LEGUMINOSAE

Genus SINDORA

SINDORA INERMIS Merr. (Fig. 9). KAYU-GÁLU.

Local names: *Kayu-gálu* (Cotabato); *pariná* (Albay); *sinsúd* (Jolo, Manukmangka Island, Sibutu Island).

KAYU-GÁLU OIL

The trunk of this species yields a resinous oil known as kayu-gálu oil. It has a pleasant, persistent odor and should be useful as a perfume oil. Locally it serves much the same purposes as the oil of supa from *Sindora supa*. It has been exported in small quantities to Singapore by Chinese traders in Zamboanga.

Sindora inermis is a tree reaching a height of about 30 meters and a diameter of about 75 centimeters. The leaves are alternate and pinnate with four to eight leaflets, which are opposite, leathery, smooth, somewhat rounded at the base, usually pointed at the tip, and from 5 to 10 centimeters in length. The flowers are borne on compound, hairy inflorescences. The fruit is flattened, somewhat inequilateral, about 7 centimeters long, and 5 centimeters wide. *Sindora inermis* is distinguished from *Sindora supa* by the fact that the fruit of *Sindora inermis* is not armed with spines as is the case with that of *Sindora supa*. This species is distributed from southern Luzon to Mindanao and Jolo.

SINDORA SUPA Merr. (Fig. 10). SUPÁ.

Local names: *Manápo, yakál-diláu, baláyong* (Tayabas); *supá* (Tayabas, Camarines, Albay, Zamboanga).

SUPÁ OIL

Oil of supa is obtained from this tree by making a cavity in' the trunk. Clover * says that a freshly cut tree will yield about 10 liters of oil. The oil is non-drying, limpid, light yellow, homogeneous, with a slight fluorescence, possesses a pleasant aromatic odor, and does not become rancid. This oil is highly prized by the Filipinos for illuminating purposes and for the treatment of skin diseases. The oil of supa can be utilized in making varnishes, paints, transparent paper, and for the adulteration of other oils.

Clover * investigated the chemical properties of the oil of supa

---

* Clover, A. M., Philippine wood oils. Philippine Journal of Science, Section A, Volume 1 (1906), page 191.

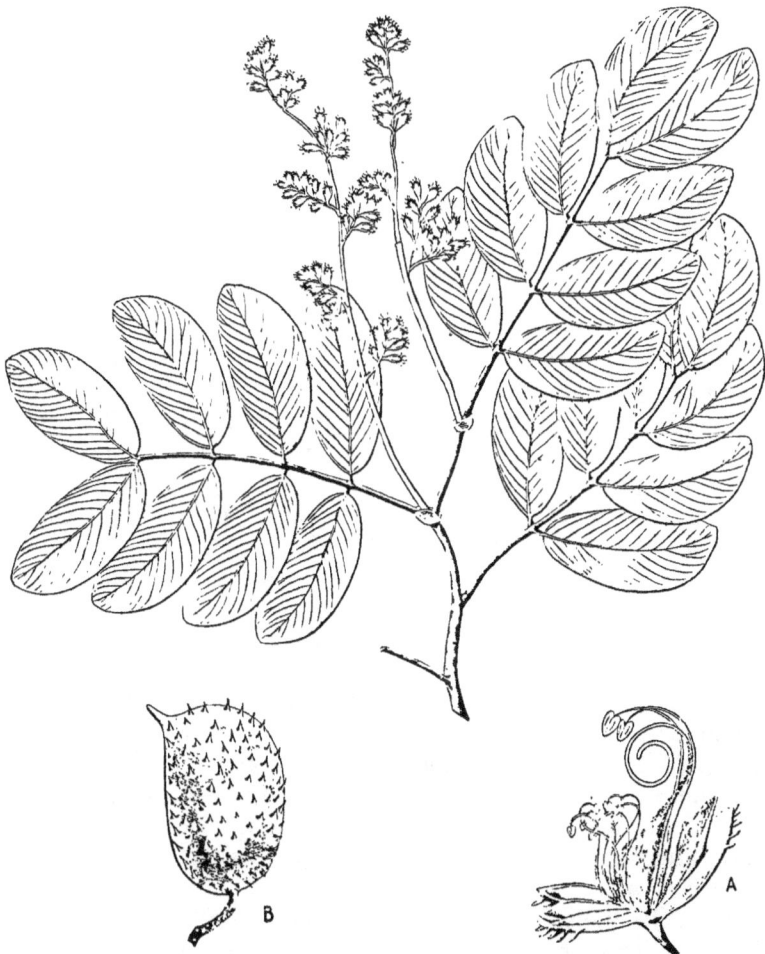

FIGURE 10. SINDORA SUPA (SUPÁ), THE SOURCE OF OIL OF SUPÁ.

and obtained the following results: Specific gravity $\frac{30}{30} = 0.9202$.
Optical rotation —31° .3 (10 centimeters, 30°). When cooled
below 20°, white crystals of a hydrocarbon were obtained. This
hydrocarbon is present to the extent of a few per cent. The oil
is soluble in ordinary organic solvents except alcohol. When exposed to the air it absorbs oxygen slowly and finally hardens.
When steam-distilled, a colorless oil is obtained. The absence
of alcoholic substances was proved by the fact that the oil is not
acted upon by sodium or phosphorous pentoxide in benzol. When
an acetic acid solution of the steam distillate was treated with
hydrochloric acid gas, cadinene hydrochloride was obtained. The
oil is therefore probably a mixture of sesquiterpenes. The non-
volatile portion of the oil which remains after distillation was
recrystallized from alcohol. Its saponification number was found
to be 64, which shows that the saponifiable matter is negligible.

Sindora supa is a tree reaching a height of 20 to 30 meters
and, in exceptional cases, a diameter of 150 to 180 centimeters.
The bole is straight, regular and without buttresses. The bark
is 7 to 10 millimeters thick, brown to nearly black in color, and
sheds in large scales. When the bark is freshly shed it exposes
pink-colored patches. The leaves are alternate and simply compound, usually with three pairs of leaflets. These are smooth,
leathery in texture, from 3.5 to 9 centimeters long, and from
2.5 to 5 centimeters wide. The fruit is a pod covered with
straight, stiff spines on the ends of which drops of sticky oil
accumulate.

The wood is hard and heavy. The heartwood is yellow or
pinkish when fresh, gradually turning to a dark-bronze color
with age. This wood was used formerly in general construction
for beams, joists, rafters, etc., and in bridge, wharf, and ship
building. It is now too highly prized for interior finish, furniture, and cabinet work, and especially flooring, to be put to
the former uses. It is an excellent wood for fine turned and
shaped tool handles, rulers and other desk supplies.

This species is intolerant of shade, occurs on limestone ridges,
and appears to be confined to a limited portion of those regions
without a distinct dry season.

Family BURSERACEAE

Genus CANARIUM

CANARIUM LUZONICUM (Bl.) A. Gray. (Figs. 11, 12).   PÍLI.
    Local names: *Alangkí* (Union); *ánteng* (Cagayan, Abra, Isabela); *ba-*
kóog (Ilocos Sur); *buláu* (Pangasinan); *malapíli* (Camarines); *pagsai-*

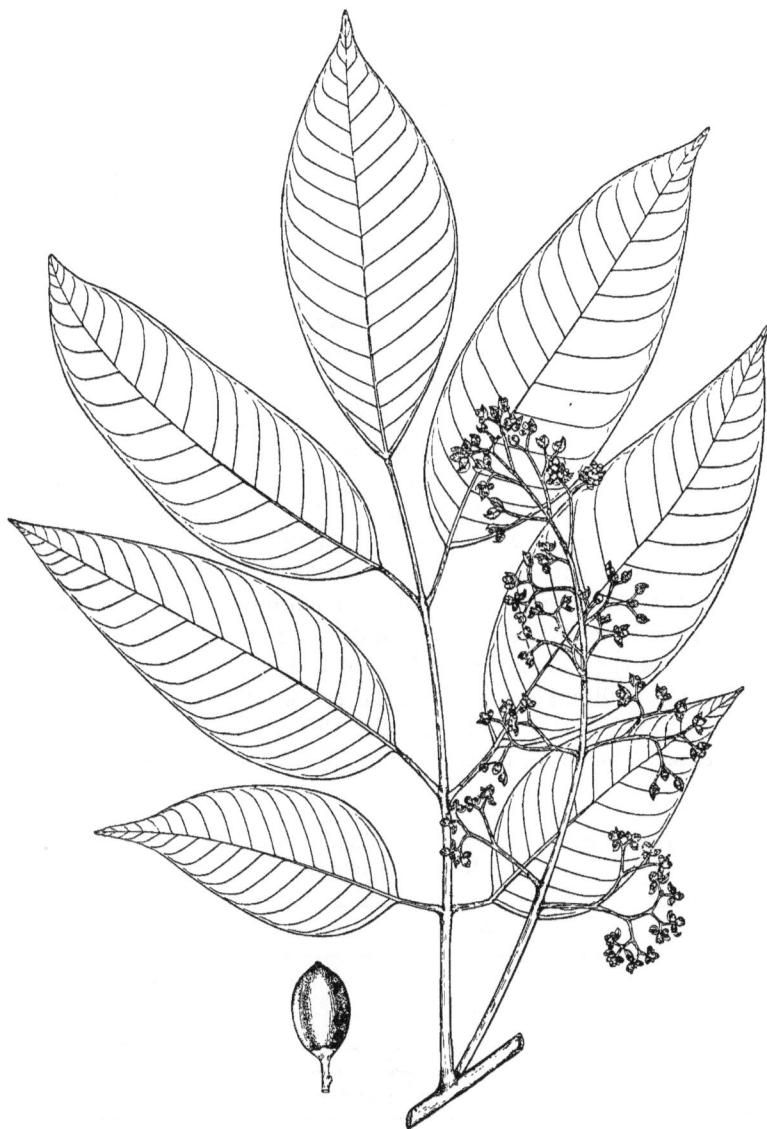

FIGURE 11. CANARIUM LUZONICUM (PILI), THE SOURCE OF MANILA ELEMI. ×⅔.

ñgin or pagsahiñgin (Rizal, Bataan); palsahiñgin (Laguna, Bataan); píli (Tayabas, Masbate, Laguna, Mindoro, Rizal, Marinduque, Tarlac, Bataan, Albay, Sorsogon); písa (Cavite); sáhing (Bataan); tugtugín (Tayabas).

MANILA ELEMI

The name elemi is a term applied to a variety of resinous products obtained from different countries and having different botanical origins. There appears, however, to be little doubt that the species concerned all belong to the family Burseraceae. The greater part of the world's supply is derived from the Philippine Islands, and is known as Manila elemi. It is obtained from the trunk of *Canarium luzonicum* and is known locally by the Spanish term brea blanca (white pitch).

Brea of the best quality is soft, sticky, opaque, slightly yellow in color, has a very agreeable resinous odor, and burns with a smoky flame. It is used locally as a varnish, for caulking boats, and for torches. As the brea is very sticky, in preparing the torches, it is usually gathered in the most convenient way possible regardless of dirt and chips, and then kneaded on the ground by beating it with a piece of wood. When enough dirt has been mixed with it to make it stiff, it is rolled into shape and wrapped in a leaf of the anahau palm (*Livistona*). Near the forest, these torches are usually sold for 1 centavo each, but in towns they are retailed for about 3 centavos each. They give a very brilliant light and burn for a long time.

Manila elemi is exported from the Philippines in considerable quantities. The exports for the past five years are given in Table 4.

TABLE 4.—*Amount and value of Manila elemi exported from the Philippines from 1914 to 1918.*

Year.	Amount.	Value.
	Kilo-grams.	*Pesos.*
1914	35,652	9,478
1915	11,380	3,781
1916	104,311	45,852
1917	78,848	29,525
1918	17,136	9,828

Some of the resin is shipped from Manila to Europe for use in preparing medicinal ointments and, to a smaller extent, in the manufacture of varnish; while much of the product is sent to China and is there used for making transparent paper

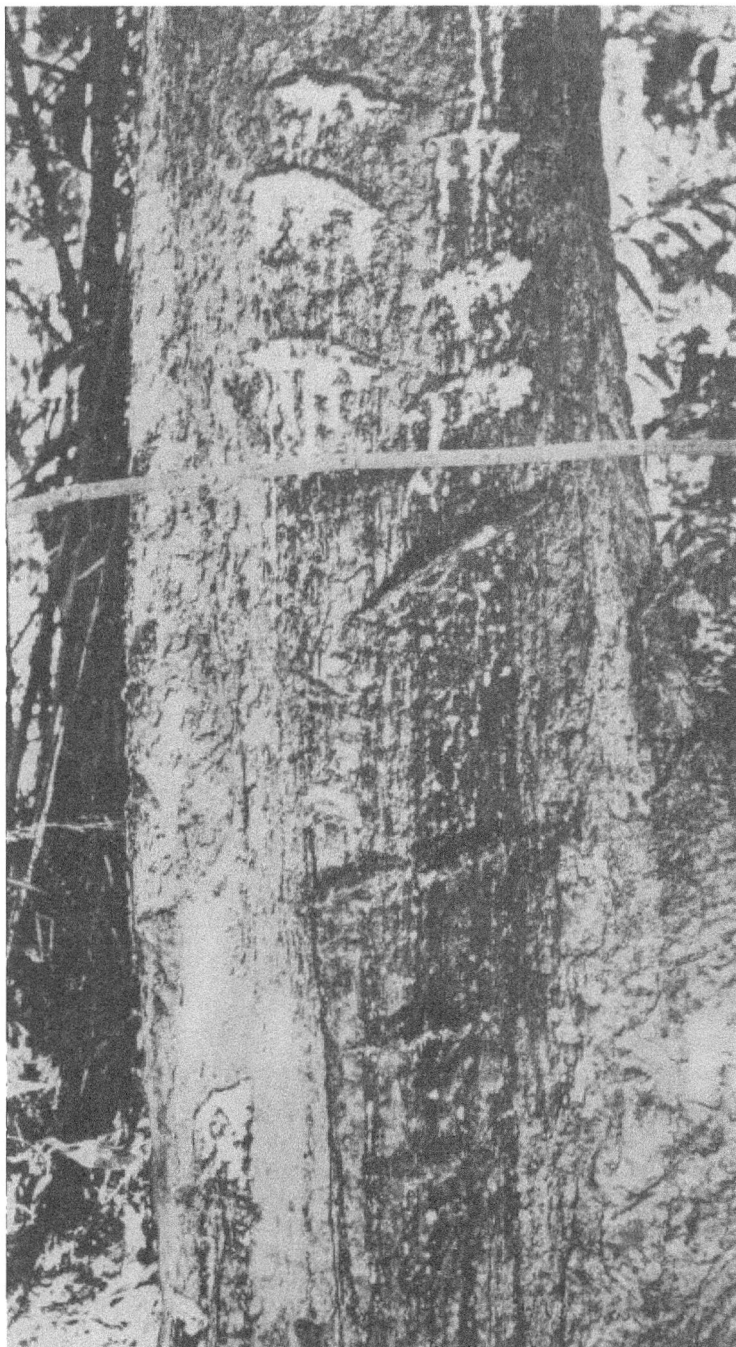

FIGURE 12. RESIN EXUDING FROM A TAPPED CANARIUM.

for window-panes, in place of glass. In America it is rarely employed medicinally.

The resin of Manila elemi is valuable as a material for preparing varnish, while the volatile oils are suitable for many purposes for which ordinary turpentine is used.

Bottler and Sabin *, in discussing elemi, say:

* * * It is not by itself made into a varnish, but is added to a variety of spirit varnishes; it makes them less brittle and more elastic. For this the various sorts of elemi are better than turpentine, because they hold their volatile oil more tenaciously. To make varnishes elastic, elemi, castor-oil, and Venetian turpentine are melted together, and this compound is added to the solution of resin.

The following formula given by Bottler and Sabin is an example of an elastic varnish containing elemi.

WHITE VARNISH SUITABLE FOR BOOKBINDERS.

	Parts.
Sandarac	6
Mastic	3
Elemi	3
Alcohol	150

Concerning the use of Manila elemi for varnish, Bacon † states:

The use of *elemi* residues with turpentine and linseed oil has not given us very satisfactory varnishes, for even with excessive quantities of driers, the varnish coat remains somewhat sticky for three or four days. This *elemi* residue, however, mixed with varying proportions of Manila copal, melted with boiled linseed oil, and properly thinned with turpentine has given us most excellent varnishes, which give a hard, brilliant, and elastic coating on wood. The use of the *elemi* resin for varnishes seems not only to give a paler and more brilliant varnish than copal alone, but renders the melting of the copal much easier. I believe this *elemi* resin distillation residue has a future as a varnish gum.

In the Philippines only one elemi gum is collected and this is obtained from *Canarium luzonicum*. When it first flows from the tree it is soft, but in the course of time hardens, the difference between the soft and the hard resin being that the latter has lost the greater part of its volatile constituents through evaporation.

In Masbate, according to Forester Zschokke, the trees are tapped at the beginning of the rainy season and the process is repeated every other day until December. The resin is collected once a month and one man can take care of from 75 to 100 trees.

* Bottler, M. and Sabin, A. H., German and American varnish making, (1912), page 21.

† Bacon, R. F., Philippine terpenes and essential oils, III. Philippine Journal of Science, Section A, Volume 4 (1909), page 100.

The trees must be visited regularly to get good returns. The resin can be gathered at almost all seasons, but towards the end of the dry season the flow is very slight. Resin is collected from the same trees·year after year. Clover * says that he has seen large-sized trees on which at least ten pounds of resin had accumulated, probably within a month. Bacon † estimates that mature trees will yield an average of 45 kilos per year. He says that he has seen as much as 32 kilos of resin on a large tree. This amount represented a two months flow.

In some localities where the resin is collected, it sells for about 50 centavos per arroba of 11.5 kilos if clean and white, but when dark for about 30 centavos. In larger towns the best quality sells for about a peso a kilo and in Manila for about 3 pesos. If the industry of collecting the resin were systematized, the cost in Manila would certainly be greatly reduced.

Bacon ‡ collected over one hundred specimens of elemi resin from individual trees. These samples of fresh elemi resin were distilled *in vacuo,* the volatile oils were then separated from the water, shaken out with dilute alkalies, dried over calcium chloride, and redistilled *in vacuo;* only the terpene fraction was collected. The terpenes were then distilled at ordinary pressure. These results verified the conclusions of Clover that the terpene oils of elemi resin obtained from different trees showed great differences in their boiling points and especially in optical rotation. For purposes of purification and identification, the various distillates of elemi resin were divided into different groups according to their boiling points. Bacon found that these distillates consisted largely of various terpenes such as alpha and beta phellandrene, dipentene, limonene, etc. He prepared various derivatives of these terpenes, such as phellandrene nitrite, dipentene tetrabromide, limonene tetrabromide, etc. Judging from Bacon's experiments, the best method for purifying elemi resin is by solution in benzene, filtering off the impurities such as bark and dirt, and distilling the filtrate. A white resin of leafy appearance is thus obtained.

Bacon investigated nine samples of carefully purified terpenes from elemi resin obtained in Gumaca, Tayabas. The results are recorded in Table 5.

* Clover, A. M., The terpene oils of Manila *elemi.* Philippine Journal of Science, Section A, Volume 2 (1907), pages 1 to 40.

† Bacon, R. F., Philippine terpenes and essential oils, III. Philippine Journal of Science, Section A, Volume 4 (1909), pages 93 to 265.

‡ Bacon, R. F., Philippine terpenes and essential oils, III. Philippine Journal of Science, Section A, Volume 4 (1909), page 93.

TABLE 5.—*Manila elemis from Gumaca, Tayabas.*

No.	N $\frac{30°}{D.}$	Boiling point.	Specific gravity, $\frac{30°}{4°}$.	A $\frac{30°}{D.}$
		Degrees.		
1	1.4674	175 -177	0.8360	116.8
2	1.4658	165 -169	0.8350	92.2
3	1.4673	175.5-178	0.8360	117.8
4	1.4672	175 -178	0.8359	111.8
5	1.4680	173 -175	0.8365	107.6
6	1.4670	175 -178	0.8358	117.9
7	1.4670	175 -178	0.8363	117.6
8	1.4660	166 -169	0.8355	90.7
9	1.4670	176 -177	0.8364	115.6

Bacon also investigated the residue left after the distillation of elemi. By the distillation of elemi *in vacuo*, he obtained from 12 to 18 per cent of terpenes and from 12 to 15 per cent of a higher-boiling oil. The distillation residue, usually amounting to about 70 per cent of the elemi, is a light-brown, transparent, solid resin, with a brilliant fracture. The elemi residue is completely and easily soluble in the cold in the following solvents: Alcohol, ether, benzol, petroleum ether, ligroin, xylol, chloroform, amyl acetate, acetone, methyl alcohol, carbon tetrachloride, ethyl acetate, turpentine, amyl alcohol, and glacial acetic acid. As previously stated, Bacon considered the residue obtained from the distillation of elemi to have important commercial possibilities as a varnish gum.

Clover * investigated the chemical properties of Manila elemi and found that:

As ordinarily gathered for commerce, the resin is soft, sticky, and opaque, has a slightly yellow color, and a very agreeable odor. It has a spicy, somewhat bitter taste. If left exposed to the air for some time, it gradually hardens throughout and finally becomes brittle. The resin dissolves readily and completely in ether, chloroform, and benzene, except for the separation of a small amount of water which it contains and also a very small amount of a white, granular substance. In acetic ester, acetone, ligroin, methyl and ethyl alcohol it does not dissolve completely unless sufficient solvent is used. With these solvents a white, crystalline residue remains which, with the use of alcohol in limited quantity, amounts to about 25 per cent of the total * * * . Very soft Manila *elemi* contains a considerable amount of water, less than 5 per cent however, while that which has collected on the tree for a length of time contains very little.

* Clover, A. M., The terpene oils of Manila elemi. Philippine Journal of Science, Section A, Volume 2 (1907), pages 1 to 40.

The volatile portion of elemi resin is called elemi oil and is usually obtained by steam-distilling the resin. Clover collected samples of elemi resin from different trees. These samples were distilled and the optical rotation, specific gravity, and refractive index of these various distillates determined. The results varied considerably. Clover concluded that the great variation found in the different oils was due to a difference in the resin obtained from different trees. The following experiments performed with a sample of Manila elemi show the general procedure followed throughout in working with this resin.

Sample II was collected near Atimonan, Tayabas, from a tree having a diameter of about 3 feet near the base and laden with unripe nuts. The sample, of which 815 grams were used, was softer than the previous one.

The first distillate at 125°, amounted to 50 grams (II, A); the second at 210° (II, B), was 123 grams; the third at 250° (II, C), was 30 grams. The terpene oil was distilled from II, B at reduced pressure and the residue added to II, C. The total terpene oil was 132 grams or 16.2 per cent; the high-boiling oil, 71 grams or 8.7 per cent.

II, A was decanted from a small amount of water which collected with it. It was then distilled twice at 36.5 millimeters, passing over the second time almost completely between 82°.5 and 83°.5; three-fourths of it distilled at almost a constant temperature or at most within 0°.25 (II, A, purified). $a\frac{30}{D} = +100°$. The product gave no test for phellandrene. With bromine in acetic acid the 104° to 105° melting limonene tetrabromide was obtained and a granular nitrosyl-chloride was also readily formed. It also gave dipentene dihydrochloride melting at 50°. It was distilled from metallic sodium, after which it boiled completely between 176° and 177°, accordingly at a slightly lower temperature than I, A, purified; however, it possessed the same odor and, so far as could be determined, was identical in all other respects.

II, C stood for over a year and was then fractionated twice at reduced pressure, whereupon about one-half of it was obtained as a light, yellowish-green product, boiling completely from 167° to 169°.5 at 35 millimeters (II, C, purified).

$$\text{Sp. gr., } \frac{30}{4} = 0.9522. \quad a\frac{30}{D} = -2°.7. \quad n\frac{30}{D} = 1.4973.$$

Clover was able to isolate various terpenes such as dextro-limonene, dextro-phellandrene, terpinene, and terpinolene from different samples of the resin.

Clover concluded that:

The combined results obtained by a careful examination of the oils obtained from 21 individual samples of resin establish the true composition of *elemi* oil so far as these samples may be considered as representative of the aggregate product. In several cases, notably in the last sample examined, substances were obtained which were not encountered in any other; it seems possible, therefore, that were the investigation continued, still others would be found in which new constituents would appear, although such cases would be rare and the substances themselves would constitute so small a proportion of the aggregate oil that they would scarcely need to be taken into account.

It is obvious that in considering Manila *elemi* or the oil obtained therefrom as products of a species, we must deal with an aggregate sample of these products; a sample derived from so great a number of individual trees that the peculiarities of the individuals disappear. If the native gatherer of resin utilizes a large number of trees and regularly removes the resin from them in small portions, the product which he places upon the market will be nearly homogeneous and a representative sample; but if he obtains his resin from a limited number of individuals his product will not be representative and, if he utilizes resin which has accumulated upon the trees in large quantity, it will not be homogeneous.

The great variation which I found at different times in the oil obtained from commercial *elemi* is readily explained. It is plain what the composition of *elemi* oil is when considered as an aggregate product; it should be remembered that to the laevo-limonene which accompanies phellandrene should be added an equal amount of dextro-limonene and the whole considered as dipentene.

Granted that we have a representative sample of resin, the composition of the oil will also be influenced by the following factors:

(1) The age of the resin.

(2) The temperature of the distillation. This factor will largely determine the proportion of the high-boiling part of the oil and will influence the composition of the terpene portion, because some of the terpenes suffer a change at higher temperatures.

(3) The length of time used in the distillation. This factor will influence only the proportion of high-boiling oil.

Yield of oil.—In the first seven samples examined considerable difference was found in the oil content. While there may be a certain amount of variation shown by the individual samples in this respect, it is thought that the differences found are more directly connected with the age of the resin. As previously noted, Schimmel & Co. state that the yield of oil is from 15 to 30 per cent. In several cases where I have examined samples of fresh, soft, resin purchased in Manila, I have always found the total yield to be from 25 to 30 per cent of the weight of the resin.

This species has been grown in plantations at Los Baños. Thirty-nine per cent of the seeds planted germinated. At the end of 7 years the trees averaged 4.37 meters in height and 4 centimeters in diameter.

Canarium luzonicum is a tree reaching a height of about 35 meters and a diameter of 1 meter or more. The leaves are pinnate, with usually three pairs of opposite leaflets and a terminal leaflet. The leaflets are smooth, pointed at the apex, rounded or obtusely pointed at the base, and from 12 to 20 centimeters in length. The flowers are fairly small and are borne on large compound inflorescences. The fruits are somewhat oval in shape, about 3 centimeters long, and contain a thick-shelled, triangular, edible nut.

This species is very abundant in the forests of Luzon and is also found in Marinduque, Ticao, Mindoro, and Masbate.

CANARIUM VILLOSUM F. Villa. (Fig. 13). PAGSAHÍÑGIN.

Local names: *Antél* (Ilocos Norte); *ánteng* (Ilocos Sur, Ilocos Norte, Zambales, Abra, Cagayan, Pangasinan, Union); *brea* (Zamboanga); *dalít* (Pangasinan); *giret* (Cagayan); *koribó* (Isabela); *milipíli* or *saong-sáong* (Cebu); *paksahíñgin* (Bataan); *pagsahíñgin* (Laguna, Mindoro, Manila, Bataan); *palsahíñgin* (Bataan, Rizal, Laguna, Batangas, Zambales, Marinduque); *patsaíñgin* (Rizal); *písa* (Abra); *sáling* (Palawan, Bataan); *sulu-saúñgan* (Negros); *tabúl* (Benguet).

PAGSAHÍÑGIN RESIN

This species yields a resin known locally as sahing.

It is used locally for fuel and light and in some cases as caulking material for bancas.

Bacon * examined the oil obtained from this resin and found that it consisted principally of paracymol. In a later publication Bacon † gives the results of further investigation:

In November, 1909, 3.5 kilos of resin were collected from one tree near Lamao, Bataan Province. The volatile oil was distilled from the resin *in vacuo* (4 to 6 millimeters) giving a total of 390 grams of oil (about 11 per cent). The latter had an odor like that obtained during a similar distillation of Manila elemi (*C. luzonicum* A. Gray), and the aqueous portion of the distillate contained a considerable amount of formic acid, although there were no visible evidences of decomposition of the resin during the distillation *in vacuo*. The oil was then distilled six times over sodium, using a column of glass beads in the neck of the distilling flask, and gave the following fractions:

Fraction No.	Weight.	Boiling point.	Refractive index, $N\frac{30}{D}$	Specific gravity, $\frac{30}{30}$	Optical rotation, $A\frac{30}{D}$
	Grams.	*Degrees.*			
1	102	154–158	1.4645	852	39.4
2	19	158–161	1.4660	851	34.7
3	45	161–165	1.4690	850	29.4
4	40	165–170	1.4730	849	21.1
5	47	170–175	1.4770	849	13.5
6	10	175–180	1.4795		

The residue was a thick, brown, viscous oil, which was attacked by sodium when an attempt was made to distill it over that metal.

Fraction No. 1 had a strong odor of pinene, and Nos. 1, 2, and 3 each

---

* Bacon, R. F., Philippine terpenes and essential oils, III. Philippine Journal of Science, Section A, Volume 4 (1909), page 94.

† Bacon, R. F., Philippine terpenes and essential oils, IV. Philippine Journal of Science, Section A, Volume 5 (1910), page 257.

readily gave large yields of pinene hydrochloride, melting at 125°. From⟨ the higher boiling fractions a very small quantity of dipentene was obtained, the tetrabromide melting at 124°.

The principal constituent of the volatile oil of this sample of the pagsainguin resin is therefore *d*-pinene. In a previous paper I have shown, from the examination of a very large number of specimens of Manila elemi from individual trees, that the terpenes found in these trees vary quite markedly from tree to tree, and that one tree usually yields but a single terpene. The same would probably seem to hold good for the pagsainguin resin, and it appears probable that these *Canarium* trees manufacture a large series of terpenes and also the parent substance of terpenes, *p*-cymol. The next step will be to study the resin from one tree for a considerable length of time, to discover whether, for example, an individual tree always gives a resin containing pinene, or whether at one time it yields a product having pinene as a constituent, at another, a resin containing phellandrene,⟨ etc. * * * The resin should be of considerable value in making clear the physiologic process of the plant in the formation of resins.

Canarium villosum is a tree reaching a diameter of 1 meter or over. The young branches, leaves, and inflorescences are more or less covered with soft brown hairs; in age, they become nearly smooth. The leaves are pinnate and from 20 to 50 centimeters long; the leaflets 7 to 15 centimeters in length, the base rounded, or somewhat heart-shaped, the apex pointed. The flowers are greenish white, hairy, and 4 to 5 millimeters long. The fruit is about 1 centimeter long and rounded in cross section. The wood is very similar to that of *Canarium luzonicum*.

This species is a native of, and confined to, the Philippines.⟨ It is widely distributed.

Family DIPTEROCARPACEAE

All species of the family Dipterocarpaceae produce more or less resin. The dipterocarps are for the most part large trees, many of them reaching a height of 50 or 60 meters. They are⟨ the dominant species in the tall, lowland forests in the Philippines and in many other parts in the Indo-Malayan region. One of the most striking peculiarities of this family is that the species occur in large numbers, the bulk of many forests being composed of one or a few species of dipterocarps. As the dipterocarps constitute about three-fourths of the total stand of timber in the Islands, it is evident that the dipterocarp resins could be collected in great quantities. The most important of these resins are baláu, a resinous oil obtained from *Dipterocarpus grandiflorus* (apítong), *Dipterocarpus vernicifluus* (pánau) and other species of *Dipterocarpus*, and a similar resin from *Anisoptera thurifera* (palosápis). Baláu is used locally to a considerable⟨ extent and has commercial possibilities.

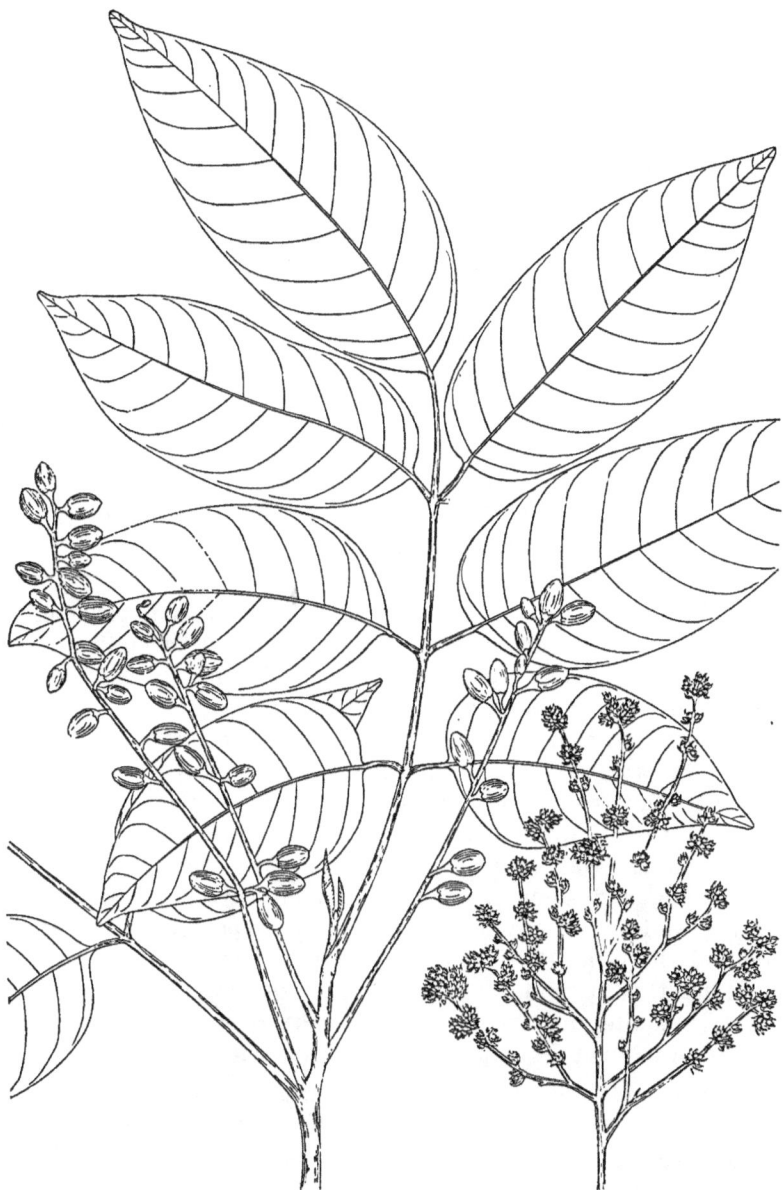

FIGURE 13. CANARIUM VILLOSUM (PAGSAHÍNGIN), THE SOURCE OF PAGSAHÍNGIN
RESIN. ×½.

The Bureau of Forestry has authentic specimens of resin
from *Hopea acuminata, Parashorea malaanonan, Pentacme con-
torta, Shorea balangeran, Shorea eximia, Shorea negrosensis,
Shorea palosapis, Shorea polysperma* and *Vatica mangachapoi*,
while Heyne reports that *Isoptera borneensis* yields resin in
small quantities.

Balau hardens only after long exposure, but most of the dipterocarp resins harden rapidly to a dry, brittle consistency
They vary from a light yellow or grayish tinge to almost black.
Very little is known of the chemical composition or possible
industrial uses of the various quick-drying dipterocarp resins.

Genus ANISOPTERA

ANISOPTERA THURIFERA Blanco. (Figs. 14, 15).   PALOSÁPIS.

Local names: *Apítong* (Sibuyan Island, Capiz); *apnít, dúung* (Abra);
bagobalóng (Samar); *bétes* or *létis* (Masbate); *dágang* (Rizal, Bulacan,
Albay, Camarines); *dágum* (Laguna, Tayabas, Albay); *dúyong* (Ilocos
Sur, Ilocos Norte); *lauán* (Rizal); *lauán putí* (Nueva Ecija); *létis* (Ticao
Island, Iloilo); *mala-átis* (Rizal); *mayápis* (Rizal, Bataan, Zambales, Nueva
Ecija, Bulacan); *palosápis* (Zambales, Pangasinan, Bataan, Nueva Ecija).

PALOSÁPIS RESIN

A resinous oil, frequently known as oil of palosapis, is obtained
from the trunk of this species. This resin is very similar to
balau from *Dipterocarpus grandiflorus*, is obtained in the same
manner, and is used for the same purposes.

Clover * says that an examination of the resinous oil from
Anisoptera thurifera (which he called mayapis) proved it to be
similar to that from *Dipterocarpus grandiflorus* and *D. vernicifluus*, but that it dried much more rapidly than either of the
latter; that it was light colored, apparently homogenous in
composition, and so viscous that it could scarcely be poured.
Heating to 100° caused it to harden, and exposure to the air
produced the same effect, changing it to a pearly, white solid.
He found that it contained 15 per cent of water and 25 per
cent of sesquiterpene oil, which could be removed by careful
distillation without decomposition. The residue was hard.

The oil redistilled at 17 millimeters, possessed the characteristic odor
of the resin, and was very light yellow in color. Boiling point, 132° to
140° (17 millimeters. Specific gravity, $\left(\frac{30°}{30}\right)$=0.9056.

Anisoptera thurifera reaches a height of 40 to 45 meters and

---

* Clover, A. M. Philippine wood oils. Philippine Journal of Science,
Volume 1 (1906), page 191.

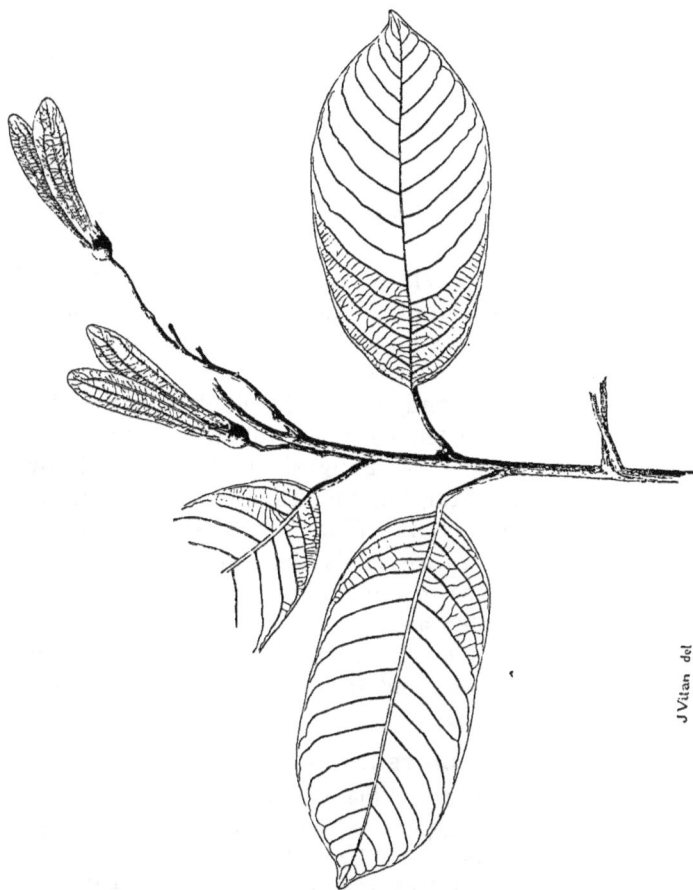

J Vitan del

FIGURE 14. ANISOPTERA THURIFERA (PALOSÁPIS), THE SOURCE OF PALOSÁPIS RESIN.

a diameter of 140 to 180 centimeters. It has a straight, regular, unbuttressed bole that is three-fifths to two-thirds of the height of the tree. The canopy is dense during the rainy season and open in the dry, at which time it changes leaves. The bark is from 15 to 25 millimeters thick; in young trees smooth and with a yellowish tinge; in older trees, especially at the base, broken into irregular patches and dirty brown in color. The bark beneath the surface has a reddish-brown color; the inner bark is granular brownish-yellow; the granular coloring being due to broken, concentric rings of yellow. The leaves are alternate, rounded at the base, pointed at the tip, from 7.5 to 16 centimeters long, and from 3 to 7 centimeters wide. The fruit is rounded, 4 to 15 millimeters in diameter, and with two wings which are 5 to 9 centimeters long, and sometimes more than a centimeter broad.

The heartwood is yellowish with rose-colored streaks and blotches or evenly rose-colored. When seasoned, the color is pale yellow with reddish or light yellowish-brown markings. It is used considerably for construction.

This species is common and widely distributed in the Philippines. It has been reported from the following localities:— Ilocos Norte, Ilocos Sur, Abra, Pangasinan, Zambales, Nueva Ecija, Bulacan, Bataan, Rizal, Laguna, Tayabas, Camarines, Albay, Sibuyan Island, Capiz, Iloilo, Ticao Island, Samar, Masbate, Zamboanga. *Anisoptera thurifera* is the commonest and best known species of the genus in the Philippines, but the wood of all is known commercially as palosapis. According to Foxworthy,* palosapis ranks about tenth in order of abundance among the Philippine woods and makes up about 1.5 per cent of the volume of the forests.   ʿ

Genus DIPTEROCARPUS

DIPTEROCARPUS GRANDIFLORUS Blanco. (Figs. 16–19).   APÍTONG.

Local names: *Anaháuon* (Camarines); *apítong* (Bataan, Cagayan, Isabela, Abra, Benguet, Zambales, Nueva Ecija, Bulacan, Laguna, Tayabas, Camarines, Albay, Mindoro, Sibuyan Island, Samar, Negros, Palawan); *baláu* (Misamis, Sibuyan Island, Negros, Capiz, Misamis, Agusan); *danlóg, létis* (Capiz); *dúen* (Isabela); *dukó* (Isabela; Apayaó); *dukó, pamalalien* (Cagayan); *hagakhák* (Sibuyan Island); *himpagtán* (Samar); *kamúyau* (Palaui Island, Cagayan); *malapáho, mayápis* (Tayabas); *pagsahíñgan* (Laguna); *pamantúlen* (Pangasinan); *pamarnisen* (Cagayan, Camarines); *pánau* (Bataan, Zambales, Rizal); *pánau verdadero* (Bulacan).

---

* Foxworthy, F. W., Philippine Dipterocarpaceae, II. Philippine Journal of Science, Volume 13 (1918), pages 163–197.

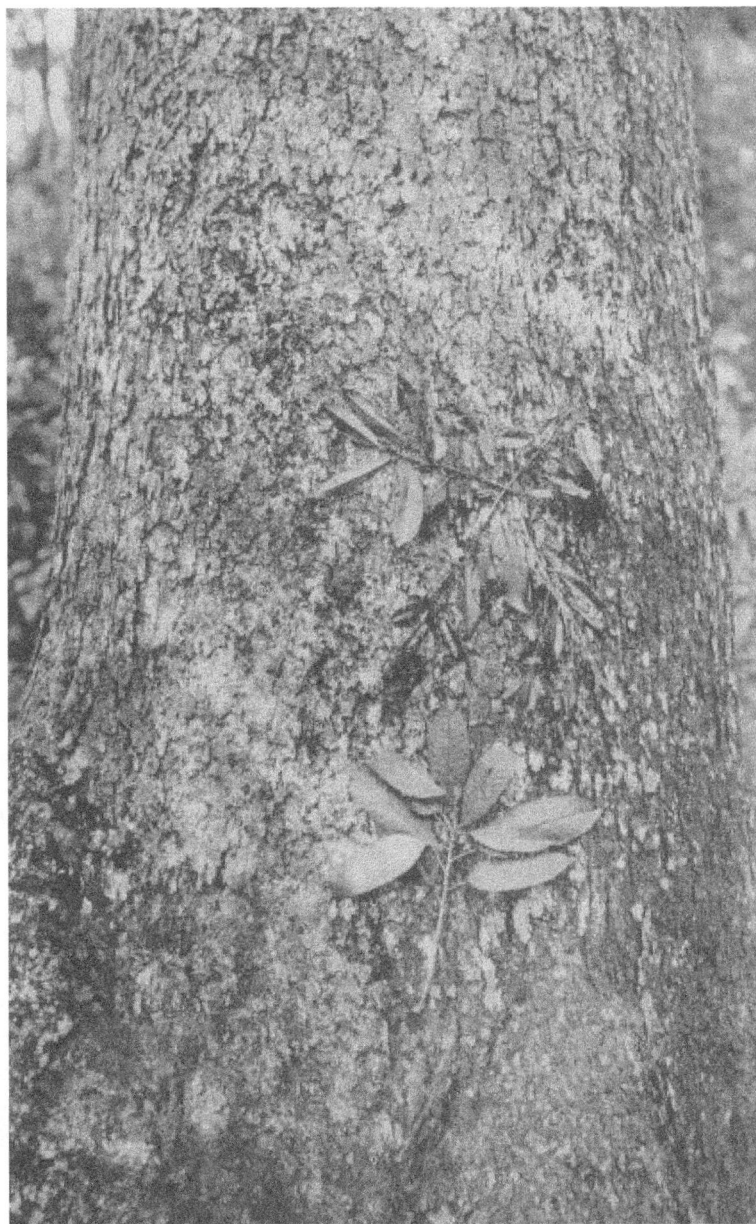

FIGURE 15. BARK AND LEAVES OF ANISOPTERA THURIFERA (PALOSÁPIS), THE SOURCE OF PALOSÁPIS RESIN.

BALÁU (APITONG) RESIN

Oil obtained from the trunk of this tree is known as baláu, and is used locally as an illuminant, for varnishing, and for caulking boats. Baláu resin used as a varnish produces a very brilliant, tough, and durable coating and according to Bacon * seems to have properties that would make its general use for varnish manufacture desirable. It has, however, the serious disadvantage of drying very slowly and, in its original state, has not yet been successfully combined with linseed oil or other dryers. Bacon, by distillation, obtained a hard, yellow, lustrous resin soluble to the extent of about 75 per cent in alcohol or turpentine, the solutions giving hard, lustrous varnish coatings. This resin dissolves completely in two volumes of linseed oil and two of turpentine, giving a varnish which dries slowly (five days) to a tough, hard coating.

Balau is collected by chopping into the tree and making a cavity where the oil can collect. Often the cuts extend halfway through the trunk. The flow may amount to more than a kilo per day. It is customary to remove the resin every few days and to apply fire to the cuts at frequent intervals. It is reported that the same tree can be tapped for a number of years. Tapping usually results in the entrance of decay organisms and the ultimate death of the tree. For this reason all trees which are tapped for balau should be cut and used for timber before the wood is destroyed.

Balau is a thick fluid when fresh, but hardens after long exposure to a semi-plastic condition. The total recorded production in 1917 was 54,080 kilos.

According to Clover † baláu consists of a solid resin, water, and a volatile oil which is present to the extent of about 35 per cent. Baláu has a feeble, characteristic odor and dissolves in the usual organic solvents except alcohol. The water which the oil contains appears to be chemically combined and is not removed easily by distillation. When distilled directly, all the water and a portion of the oil passes over below 260°. A sample was distilled under diminished pressure (40 mm.) at 151° to 154°. The optical rotation of this fraction was 78°.5 (10 centimeters, 30°). The specific gravity was $\frac{30}{30}$ =0.9127. It had

---

* Bacon, R. F., Philippine terpenes and essential oils, III. Philippine Journal of Science, Section A, Volume 4 (1909), page 93.

† Clover, A. M., Philippine wood oils. Philippine Journal of Science, Section A, Volume 1 (1906), page 195.

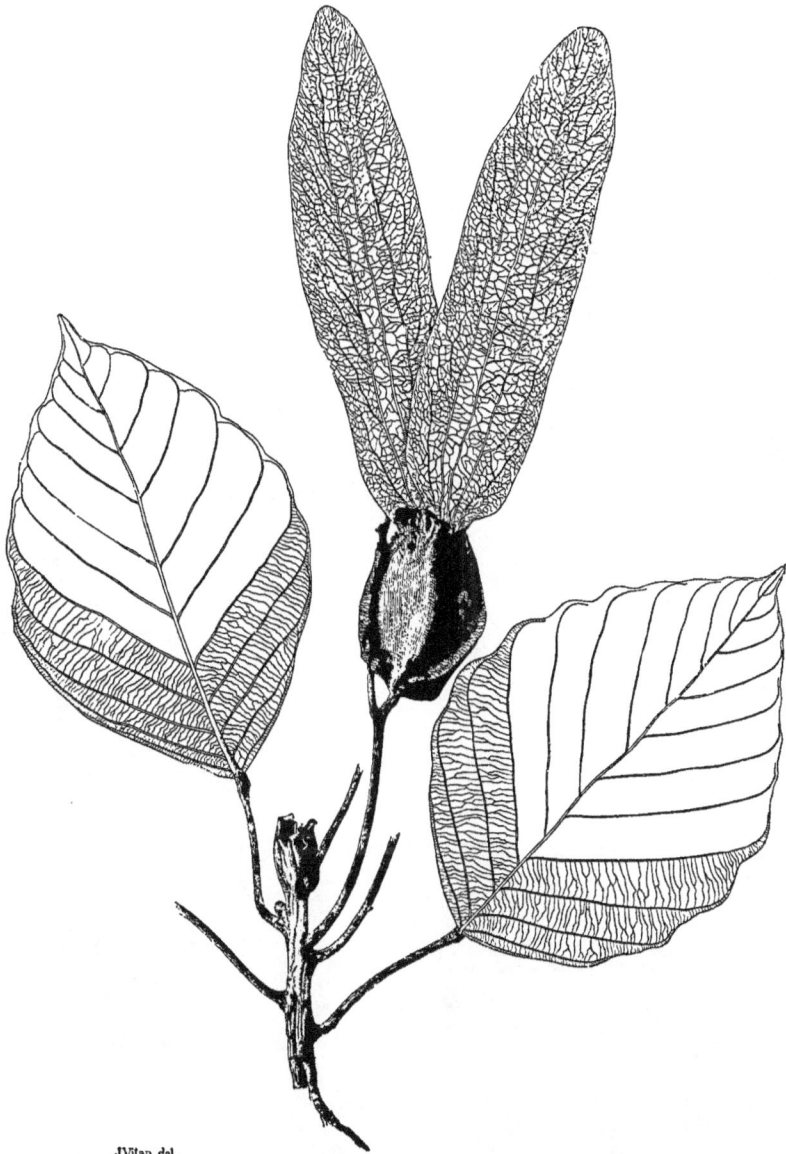

J.Vilan del.

FIGURE 16. DIPTEROCARPUS GRANDIFLORUS (APÍTONG), A SOURCE OF BALÁU.

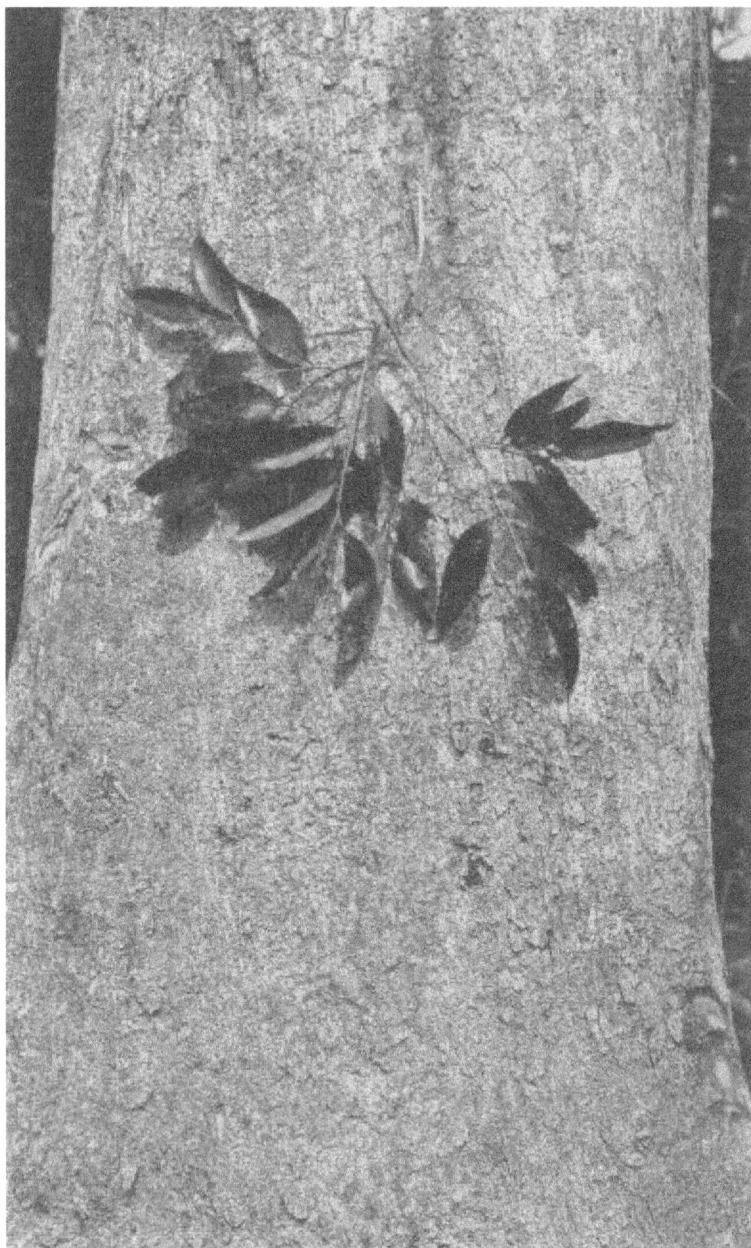

FIGURE 17. BARK AND LEAVES OF DIPTEROCARPUS GRANDIFLORUS (APÍTONG), A SOURCE OF BALÁU.

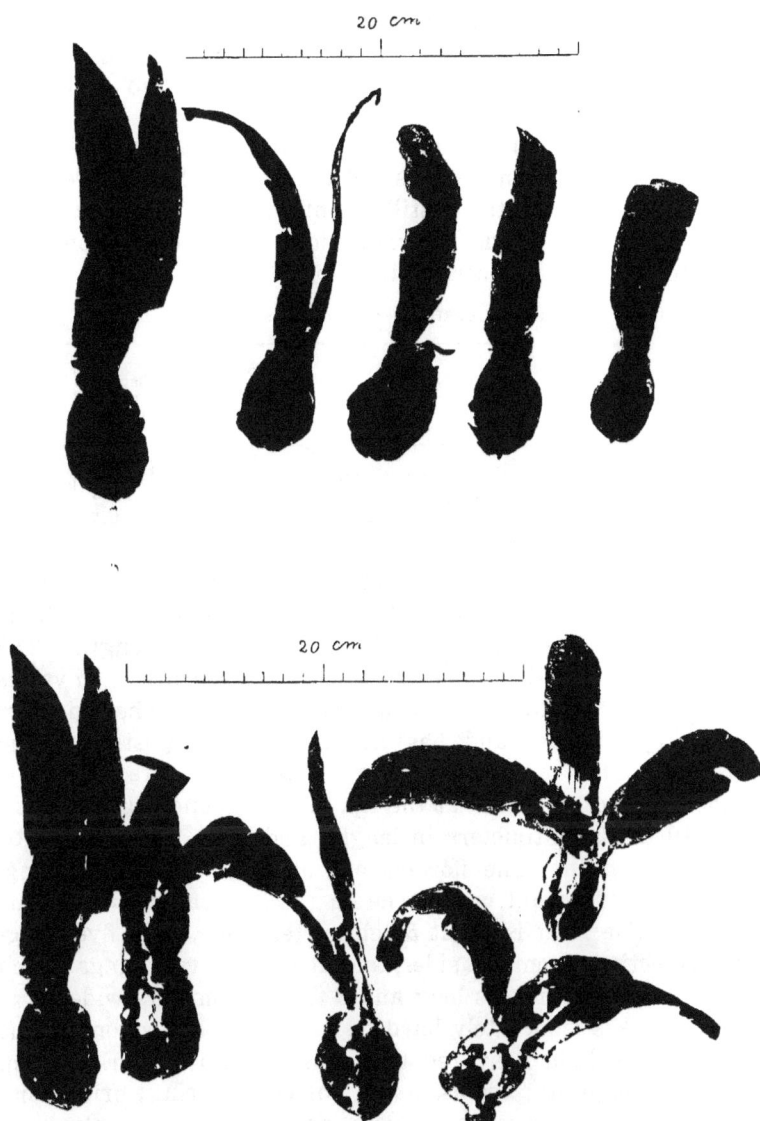

FIGURE 18. FRUITS OF DIPTEROCARPUS GRANDIFLORUS (APITONG).

a light yellow color and the characteristic odor of baláu. Treatment with sodium shows that it contains no alcoholic substances. Although it reacts with halogen acids, it was not possible to separate out a crystalline substance such as a hydrochloride. As the range in the boiling point of baláu is considerably greater than that of a pure chemical compound, it is probably a mixture of sesquiterpenes.

Bacon * performed a number of experiments to determine the solubility of baláu in various solvents. He also distilled the resin and separated the distillate into various fractions. Dr. M. V. del Rosario made determinations on these fractions and obtained the results recorded in Table 6.

TABLE 6.—*Constants of fractions of Baláu.*

No.	Specific gravity. $\frac{20°}{4.°}$	Index number.	Saponification number.	Acid number.
1	0.9089	268.3	4.01	1.8
2	0.8882	192.1	10.7	23.0
3	0.9387	120.9	12.75	18.0

Dipterocarpus grandiflorus reaches a height of from 40 to 45 meters and a diameter of 180 centimeters. The bole is straight and regular and from 25 to 30 meters in length. The bark is from 6 to 8 millimeters thick, and is brittle. It varies in color from a brown gray to a light gray. It is shed in large scroll-shaped plates and has numerous corky pustules. The inner bark has a reddish color. The leaves are alternate, leathery, smooth, pointed at the tip, usually rounded at the base, from 19 to 30 centimeters in length, and from 9.5 to 17 centimeters in width. The flowers are about 5 centimeters long, rose-colored, fragrant, and borne on racemes having about four flowers. The fruit is about 5 centimeters long, with five wing-like projections from the sides, and at one end two wings which are 14 to 23 centimeters long and 3 to 5 centimeters wide.

The wood is moderately hard to hard, stiff, and strong. The heartwood is light ashy red to reddish brown or dark brown. It is used for posts; beams, joists, rafters; flooring; bridge and wharf constructions except piles; wagon beds; ship planking, barges and lighters; ties, paving blocks, mine timbers; cheap and medium-grade furniture.

---

* Bacon, R. F., Philippine terpenes and essential oils, III. Philippine Journal of Science, Section A, Volume 4 (1909), page 93.

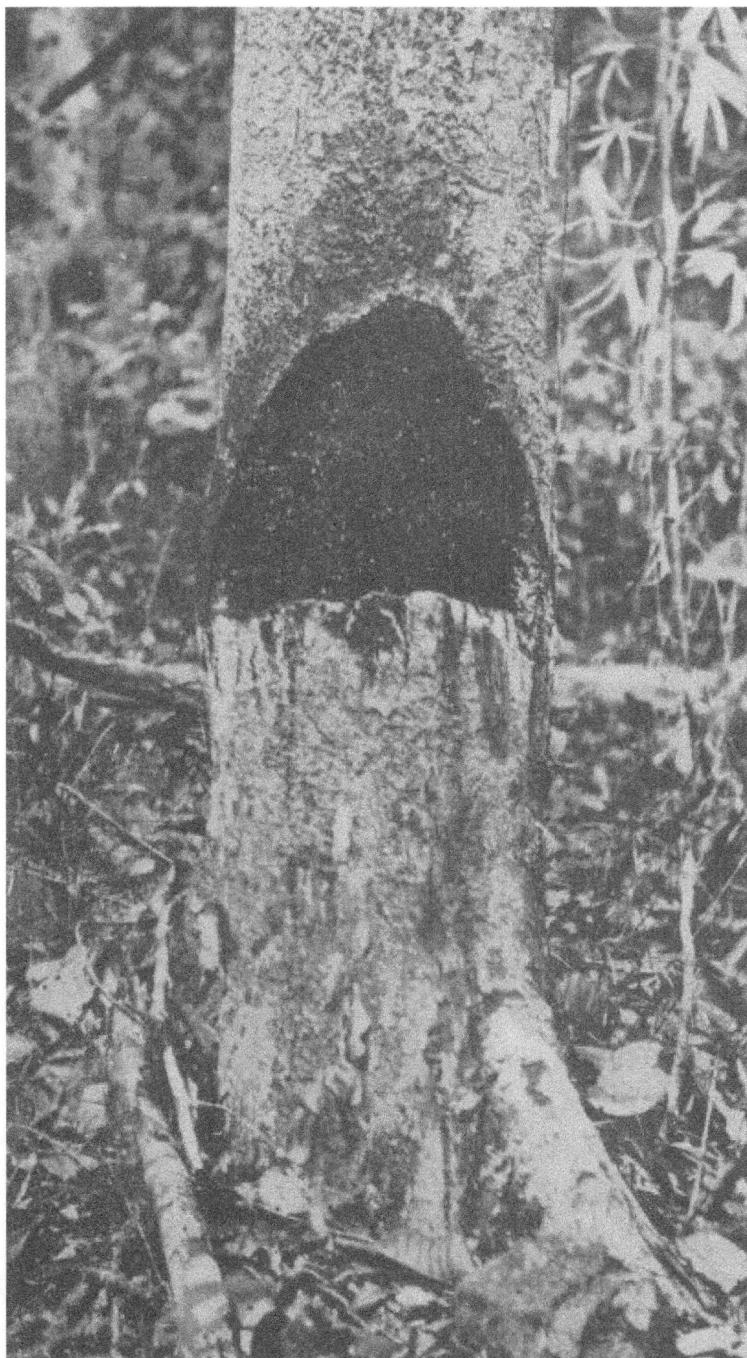

FIGURE 19. DIPTEROCARPUS GRANDIFLORUS (APITONG) BOXED FOR RESIN.

Apitong is the most generally used construction wood in the Islands. It is apparently impossible to distinguish commercially between the wood of the different species of *Dipterocarpus* and that of all the species known commercially as apitong. Apitong is the most abundant wood in the Philippine Islands, composing, according to Foxworthy,* 20 per cent of the volume of our commercial forests.

Dipterocarpus grandiflorus is found throughout the Philippine Archipelago, and has been reported from the following localities: Palaui Island, Cagayan, Isabela, Apayao, Benguet, Ilocos Sur, Pangasinan, Abra, Nueva Vizcaya, Nueva Ecija, Zambales, Bataan, Bulacan, Rizal, Laguna, Tayabas, Camarines, Mindoro, Capiz, Sibuyan Island, Albay, Samar, Negros, Palawan, Misamis, and Agusan. It is especially plentiful in regions where the dry season is pronounced.

DIPTEROCARPUS VERNICIFLUUS Blanco. (Figs. 20–22).   PÁNAU.

Local names: *Afú* (Ilocos Norte); *apítong* (Mindoro, Polillo, Bataan, Tayabas, Marinduque, Leyte, Laguna, Samar); *baláu* (Rizal, Zamboanga); *dúen, lamílan* (Isabela); *gan-án* (Camarines); *kalusúban* (Ilocos Sur); *kamúyau, kurimau, pagsaíñgin, pamarnísen* (Cagayan); *lauán* (Negros, Rizal, Nueva Ecija); *lipót* or *lipús* (Agusan); *lipús* (Surigao); *malapáho* (Polillo); *matatalína* (Zamboanga); *padsahíñgin* (Laguna); *pamantúlen* (Pangasinan); *pánau* (Rizal, Palawan, Bataan, Zambales, Bulacan, Pangasinan, Davao, Cotabato, Cagayan, Laguna, Pampanga, Tayabas, Nueva Ecija.)

BALÁU (PANÁU) RESIN

Oil obtained from the trunk of this species is very similar to baláu from *Dipterocarpus grandiflorus*, is used for the same purposes, and is regularly called baláu. This oil is also known as oil of pánau, and sometimes as malapaho.

Clover,† who investigated the chemical properties of oil of pánau states that the method of obtaining this oil from the tree is the same as that used in the case of baláu. It is reported that a gallon per day is sometimes obtained. The fresh resin is a white, viscous, sticky fluid having a characteristic odor by which it is distinguished from similar products. When exposed to the air, oxygen is absorbed and the color gradually turns brown. It hardens very slowly when exposed in a thin film. It is insoluble in water, but dissolves in ether or chloroform with the separation of water. When distilled with a free flame it acts

---

* Foxworthy, F. W., Philippine Dipterocarpaceae, II. Philippine Journal of Science, Section C, Volume 13 (1918), page 163.

† Clover, A. M., Philippine wood oils. Philippine Journal of Science, Section A, Volume 1 (1906), page 198.

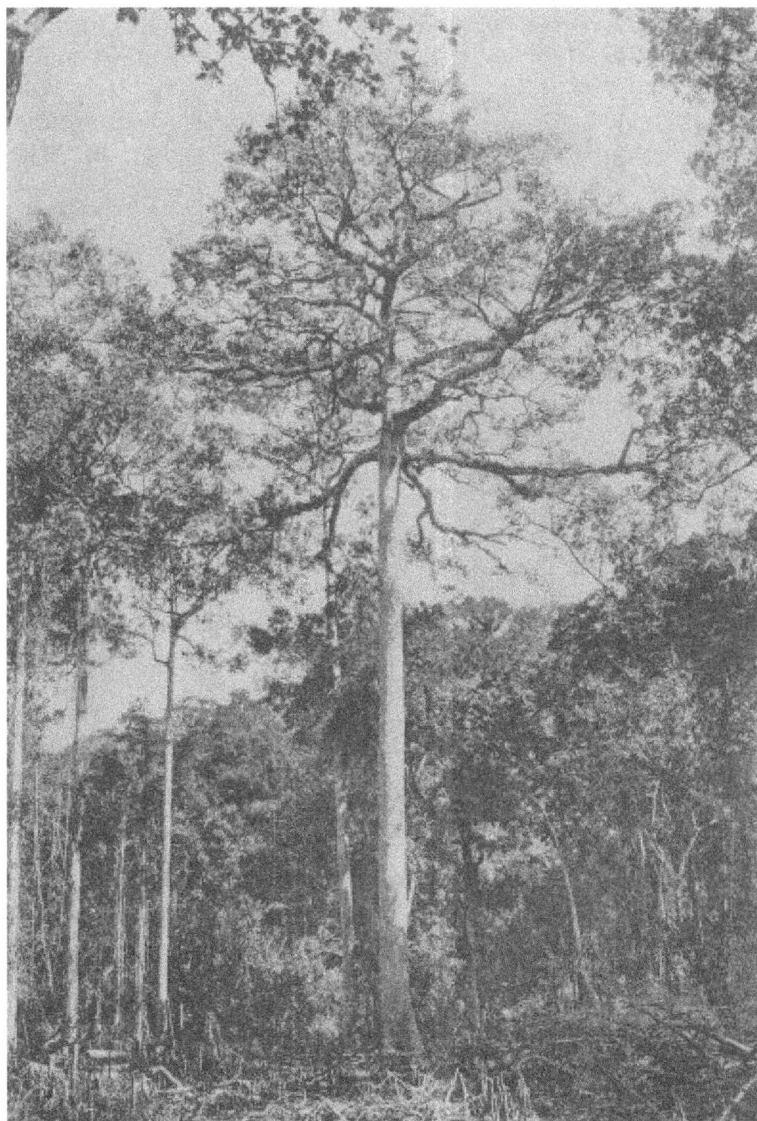

FIGURE 20. DIPTEROCARPUS VERNICIFLUUS (PÁNAU), A SOURCE OF BALÁU.

like baláu and yields about 25 per cent of water, 35 per cent of oil, and 40 per cent of solid residue. It probably consists of water, sesquiterpene oils, and solids.

Dipterocarpus vernicifluus reaches a height of 40 to 45 meters and a diameter of 160 to 180 centimeters. The bole is straight, regular, and reaches a length of 28 to 32 meters. It usually has very prominent buttresses. The bark is from 5 to 8 millimeters thick, light brown to gray in color, scaling in large patches, and is covered with numerous corky pustules. The inner bark is brown to reddish brown and stringy in texture. The young stems and the midrib and secondary nerves of the leaves are covered with long hairs. The leaves are alternate, leathery, pointed at the tip, rounded at the base, from 10 to 23 centimeters long, and 6 to 13 centimeters wide. The flowers are about 4 centimeters long, white, tinged with pink, and very fragrant. The fruits are rounded, about 1.5 centimeters in diameter and bear two long wings which are about 12 centimeters in length and 2 or 3 centimeters in breadth. The wood is very similar to that of *Dipterocarpus grandiflorus* and has the same uses.

This species abounds in regions with a pronounced dry season and has been reported from the following localities: Cagayan, Isabela, Ilocos Norte, Ilocos Sur, Pangasinan, Zambales, Nueva Ecija, Pampanga, Bulacan, Bataan, Rizal, Laguna, Tayabas, Camarines, Marinduque, Polillo, Negros, Samar, Leyte, Palawan, Misamis, Surigao, Agusan, Davao, Cotabato, and Zamboanga.

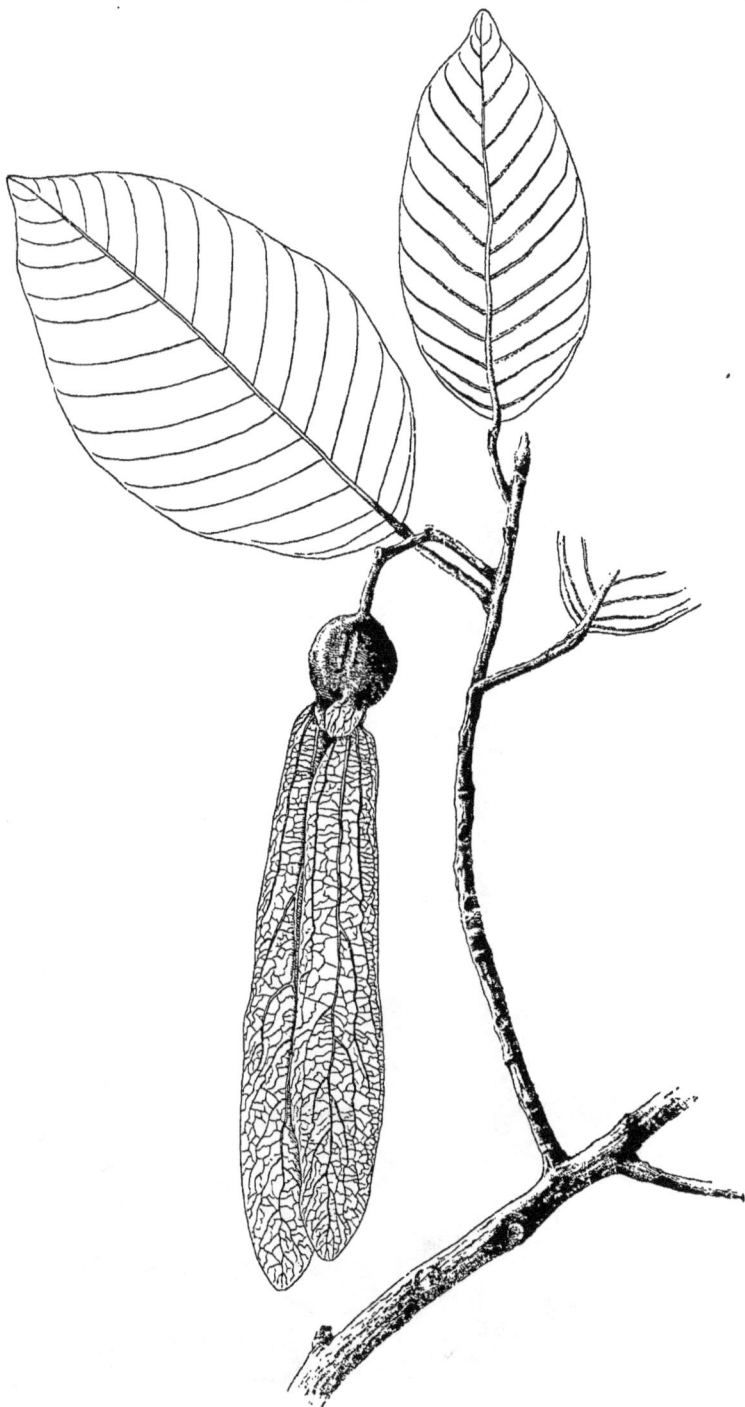

J Vilan del.

FIGURE 21. DIPTEROCARPUS VERNICIFLUUS (PÁNAU), A SOURCE OF BALÁU.

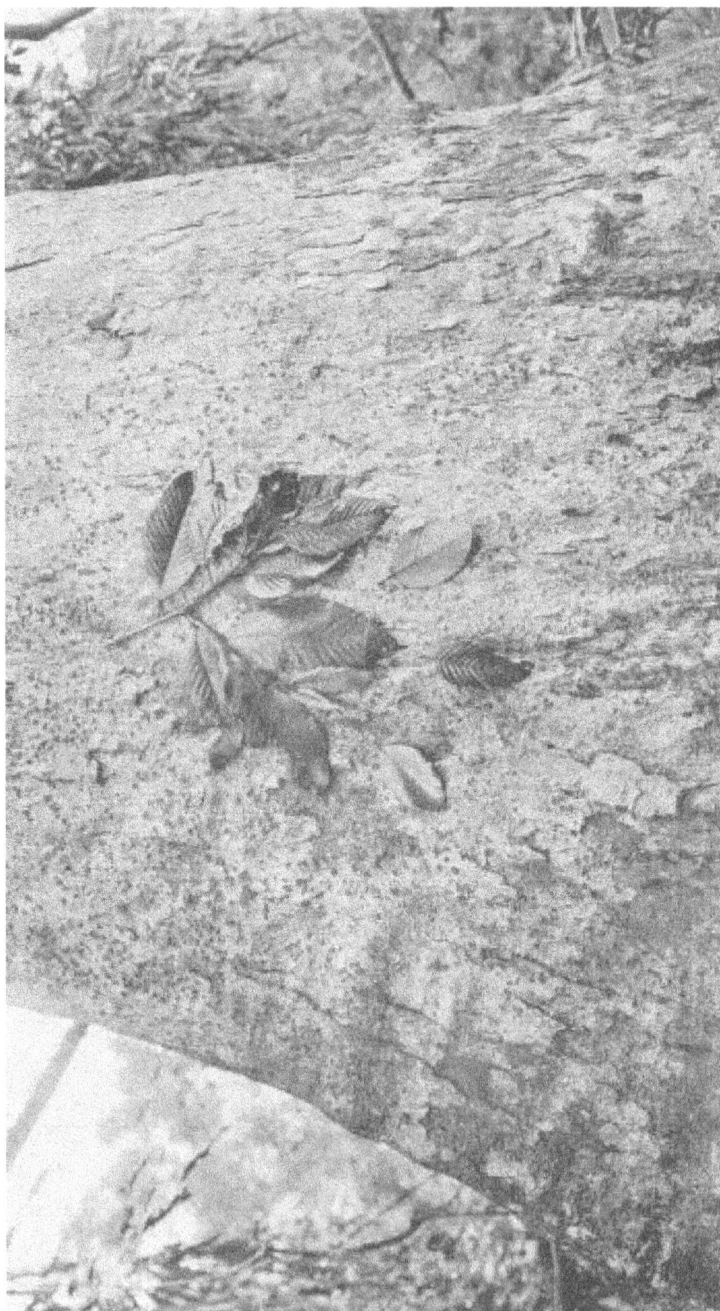

FIGURE 22. BARK AND LEAVES OF DIPTEROCARPUS VERNICIFLUUS (PANAU), A SOURCE OF BALAU.

GUMS

Gums are amorphous substances which exude from plants or which may be extracted by solvents. The true gums, such as acacia and tragacanth, have the property of either dissolving in water or taking up a sufficient amount of water to become glutinous and form a sticky liquid (mucilage). There are, however, a number of well-known substances like rubber and gutta-percha, which resemble the true gums, but are insoluble in water. Substances of this nature are obtained from plants which have capillary tubes containing a milky juice. This juice (latex) may occur in the stems, leaves, or roots. The latex appears to be an emulsion which contains a number of substances in varying proportions. An idea of the composition of one of these milky juices may be obtained from the following figures * which represent the analysis of the latex of *Hevea braziliensis*, the plant from which para rubber is obtained.

	Per cent.
Water	55.0
Rubber	38.5
Proteins	3.0
Resins	3.0
Mineral matter	0.5

The latex may be obtained by making incisions in the trunk of the tree. This cuts the latex tubes and allows the milky juice to exude. The juice thus obtained is collected in small vessels and may be coagulated in various ways, such as by smoking or by treatment with a salt solution. The latex may also be extracted by other mechanical or chemical methods.

The most important substances produced in the Philippines which may be classified as gums are rubber and gutta-percha. The wild rubber is small in amount, and the native plants do not appear to offer any prospect for a considerable industry. The southern Philippines seem, however, to be well suited for the production of plantation rubber, and the rates of growth of *Hevea braziliensis* in this region compare favorably with rates elsewhere.†

---

* Rogers, A., Industrial chemistry, 1915, page 704.

† Yates, H. S., The growth of Hevea braziliensis in the Philippine Islands. Philippine Journal of Science, Volume 14 (1919), pages 501–523.

In the Philippines very little rubber has yet been planted, despite the fact that the United States is the world's greatest consumer of crude rubber. The imports of crude rubber into the United States for the fiscal year ending June 30, 1917, were 151,533,505 kilos valued at ₱378,657,348.‡ The imports from the British and Dutch East Indies for the same period were 82,468,900 kilos valued at ₱208,451,104. At the present time practically all the plantation rubber produced in the Philippines is grown on one plantation in the Island of Basilan. Several other plantations are, however, beginning to produce rubber.

Large quantities of gutta-percha have been collected in the southern Philippines, and at the present time gutta-percha, obtained from wild species, is still being exported. However, as in the case of rubber, no very considerable industry can be expected until the trees are grown in plantations.

The next most promising Philippine gums would seem to be those which form the basis of chewing gum. Two native species of *Artocarpus* appear worthy of note in this respect, while *Achras sapota* (chico), the source of gum chicle, is grown extensively throughout the Archipelago for its edible fruits. Gum chicle is exported in enormous quantities from Mexico to the United States, where it is the principal substance used in the manufacture of chewing gum. In the Philippines this product has apparently never been collected.

Family ORCHIDACEAE

Genus GEODORUM

GEODORUM NUTANS (Presl) Ames.

Local names: *Bandabok* (Palawan); *cebollas del monte* (Cavite); *kula* (Manila); *lubi-lubi* (Negros).

GEODORUM NUTANS GUM

The tuberous roots contain a substance which is used as a glue, especially in cementing together parts of mandolins, guitars, and other musical instruments. In preparing the glue the rhizomes are first cooked and then finely grated. Glue thus prepared is said to have great tenacity.

Several other Philippine orchids are used for the same purpose.

Geodorum nutans is a terrestrial orchid with somewhat fleshy underground roots. It reaches a height of 70 centimeters. The

‡ India Rubber World, Volume 57 (1917), page 59.

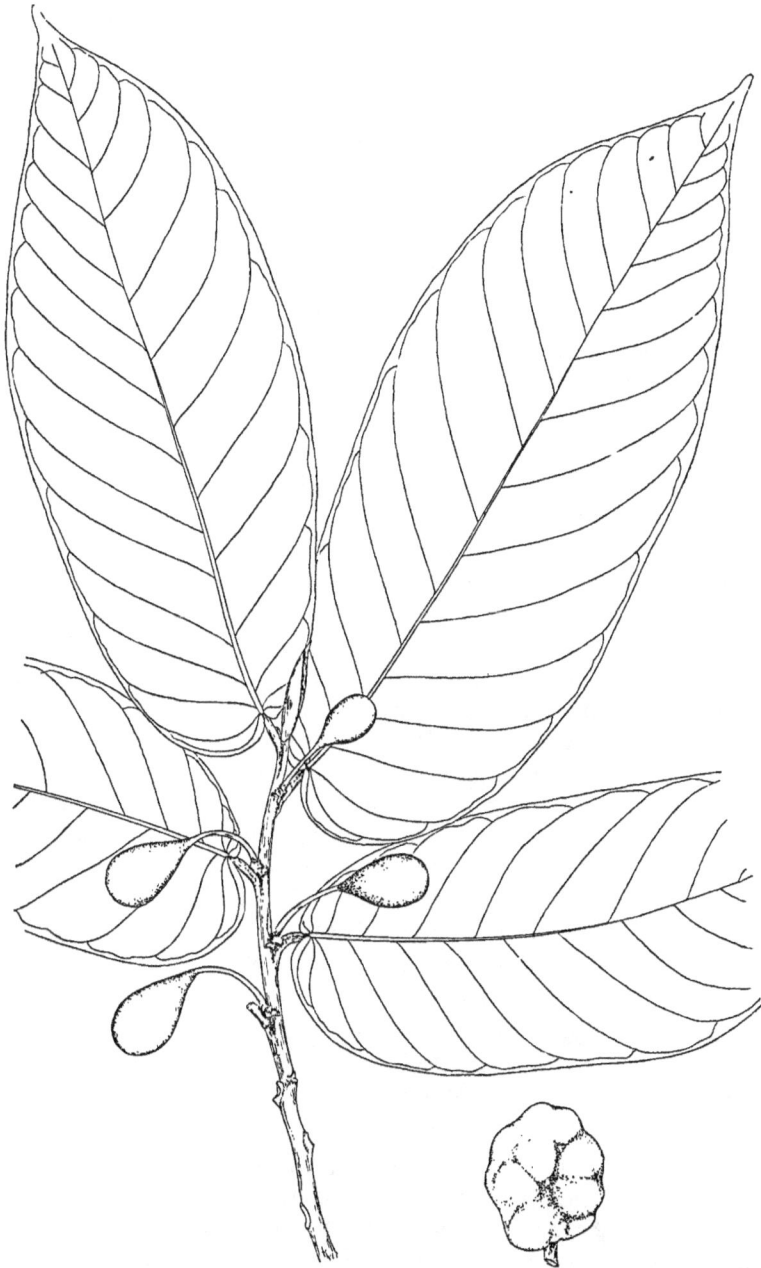

FIGURE 23. ARTOCARPUS CUMINGIANA (ANUBING), A SOURCE OF CHEWING GUM. X⅓.

shoot bears two or four large leaves, which are variable in size. The leaves are rather narrow, pointed, and up to 35 centimeters in length and 7 centimeters in width. The flowering shoots are 20 to 25 centimeters in length and leafless. The flowers are pale pink to purple, about 1 centimeter long and numerous.

This species is widely distributed in the Philippines and is also found in Formosa. It occurs particularly in thickets and open places.

Family MORACEAE

Genus ARTOCARPUS

ARTOCARPUS CUMINGIANA Tréc. (Fig. 23).   ANUBÍNG.

Local names: *Anubíng* (Nueva Ecija, Tarlac, Zambales, Rizal, Laguna,' Tayabas, Camarines, Sorsogon, Mindoro, Nueva Ecija, Sibuyan); *anubling* or *kanubling* (Camarines, Albay, Sorsogon); *bayukó, isís* (Negros, Iloilo); *kalauáhan* (Bontoc); *kamandág* (Cagayan); *koliúng* (Abra); *kúbi* (Tayabas, Mindoro, Masbate, Ticao, Negros, Surigao); *obién* or *ubién* (Abra, Ilocos Sur, Isabela, Benguet, Union).

ANUBÍNG GUM

The latex of this species would appear to be promising material for chewing gum.

This species has been grown in plantations at Los Baños. Two separate lots of seeds were planted. In one case the percentage of germination was 61.7 and in the other 28.7. At the end of 7 years the average rate of growth was 2.5 meters.

Artocarpus cumingiana is a tree reaching a height of about 30 meters and a diameter of about 100 centimeters. The leaves are alternate, hairy, pointed or slightly heart-shaped at the base, and average 20 centimeters long, and 10 centimeters wide. The petioles are 1 to 2 centimeters long. The male heads are pear-shaped and 1 to 2 centimeters long. The female heads are rounded and nearly 2 centimeters in diameter.

This species is distributed from northern Luzon to Mindanao.

ARTOCARPUS ELASTICA Reinw. (Fig. 24).   GUMÍHAN.

Local names: *Antipólo* (Tayabas, Samar); *gumíhan* (Camarines, Albay, Sorsogon); *tugúp* (Surigao, Davao).

GUMÍHAN GUM

The latex of this tree hardens into a somewhat brittle substance resembling in color and consistency the stick chewing gum put on the market years ago, before it was blended with sugar and flavored. As far as is known, the gum of *Artocarpus elastica* has not been collected in quantity nor has any analysis been made of it. The latex of some species of *Artocarpus* is used locally in compounding bird lime.

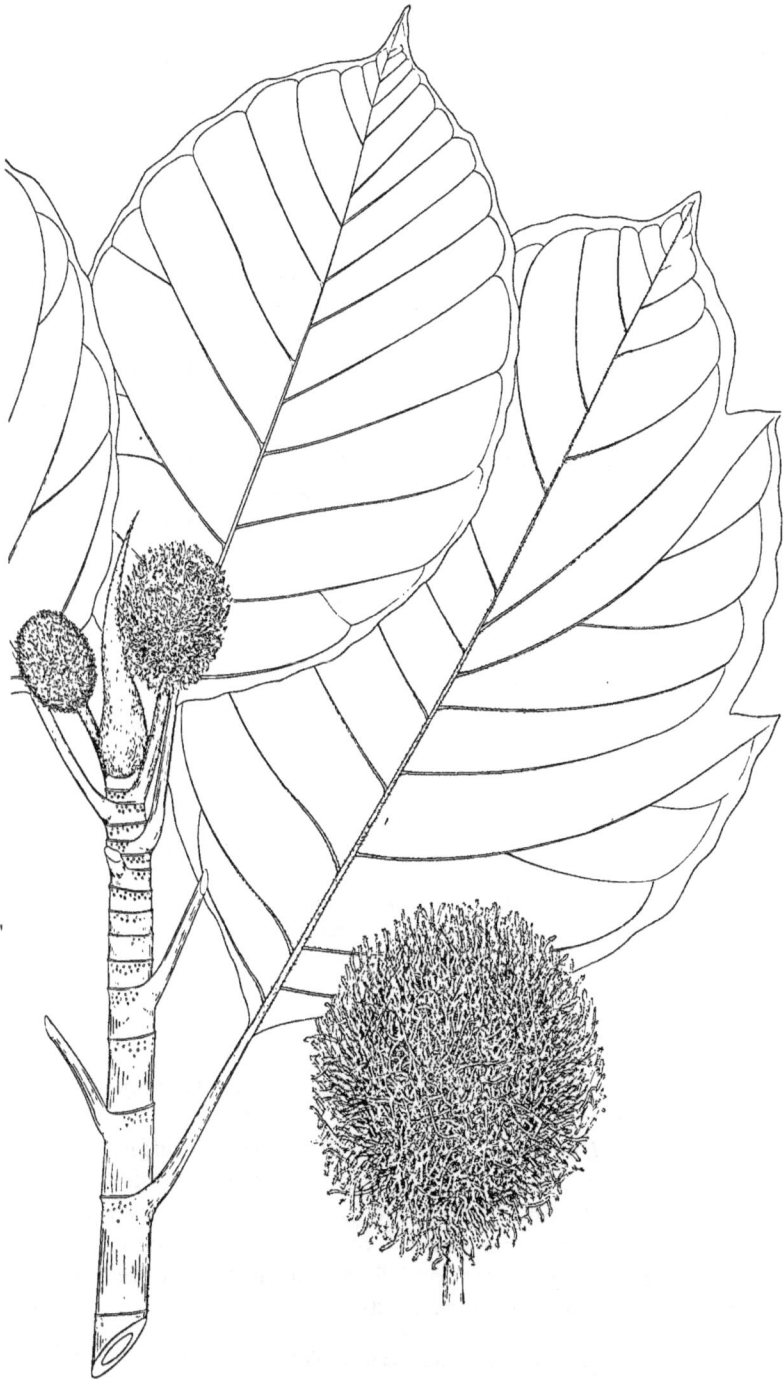

FIGURE 24. ARTOCARPUS ELASTICA (GUMiHAN), A SOURCE OF CHEWING GUM. $\times \frac{1}{2}$.

Heyne * reports that oil from the seeds of *Artocarpus elastica* is used in cooking and as a hair oil.

Artocarpus elastica is a stately tree with trunks 60 to 90 centimeters in diameter. The leaves are alternate, crowded, obtuse at both ends, occasionally lobed towards the apex, the larger ones 20 to 30 centimeters wide, and 60 to 90 centimeters long. The male spikes are cylindrical, oblong, soft or spongy, and yellowish. The female heads are somewhat rounded or elliptical. The fruit is heavy, at least 10 centimeters long, and covered with brownish, hairy appendages. The seeds are embedded in whitish, more or less gummy pulp of a delicious tart flavor. They resemble peanuts, and when roasted have a similar flavor.

There are about twenty species of the genus *Artocarpus*, all having latices which resemble those of anubing and gumihan, and which are used for various purposes such as making birdlime and other sticky substances.

Family LEGUMINOSAE

Genus ACACIA

ACACIA FARNESIANA Willd.   ARÓMA.

The gum of this species is mentioned under the heading of essential oils.

Genus SESBANIA

SESBANIA GRANDIFLORA Pers.   KATÚRAI.

Local names: *Diana* (Davao); *katúri* (Pampanga, Tayabas); *katúdai* (Ilocos Norte and Sur, Abra, Nueva Vizcaya, Pangasinan, Union); *katúrai* (Cagayan, Pangasinan, Tarlac, Bulacan, Zambales, Bataan, Rizal, Tayabas, Manila, Batangas, Laguna, Mindoro, Camarines, Zamboanga); *gauai-gáuai* (Manila, Camarines, Albay, Sorsogon, Capiz, Negros); *gaui-gáui* (Guimaras Island).

KATÚRAI GUM

This species produces a clear gum used locally as a substitute for gum arabic. The flowers and young fruits are cooked and eaten as vegetables.

Sesbania grandiflora is a tree 5 to 10 meters in height. The leaves are alternate, 20 to 30 centimeters long, and pinnate with 20 to 40 pairs of leaflets, which are 2.5 to 3.5 centimeters long. The flowers are white and from 7 to 9 centimeters long. The pods are 20 to 60 centimeters long, 7 to 8 millimeters wide, somewhat curved, and contain many seeds.

---

* Heyne, K., De Nuttige Planten van Nederlandsch-Indië, Volume 2 (1916), page 49.

This species is not uncommon in cultivation in the Philippines, and is half wild.

Family EUPHORBIACEAE

Genus MACARANGA

MACARANGA TANARIUS Muell-Arg.   BINÚÑGA.

Local names: *Alañgabun, anabun* (Bagobo); *bagambáng, ma-ásim* (Rizal); *bilúa* (Pampanga); *bilúan, binúñgan, malabúñga, biluán-laláki* (Bataan); *bilúñga* (Tayabas); *biñg-úa* (Nueva Vizcaya); *binúñga* (Bataan, Bulacan, Rizal, Laguna, Camarines, Polillo, Mindoro, Guimaras Island, Negros, Palawan); *binuga, luñgakan,* (Davao); *gamu, sámuk* (Cagayan); *ginabang* (Benguet); *labauel* (Lepanto); *lagau* (Bisaya); *lagaon, ligabon* (Manobo); *malabúñga* (Mindanao); *mindáng* (Camarines); *minúñga* (Agusan); *sámak* (Ilocos Norte, Abra, Camiguin Island).

BINÚÑGA GUM

A glue used for fastening together the parts of musical instruments such as guitars, violins, etc., is obtained from the bark of this tree. The bark is tapped by V-shaped incisions, and the sap collected and used shortly afterwards. It is said that if the sap is allowed to stand until it becomes sticky, it is worthless for the above-mentioned purposes. Heyne [*] mentions a similar use in Java.

Macaranga tanarius is a small tree reaching a height of 4 to 8 meters. The leaves are alternate, 10 to 25 centimeters long, shield-shaped, with the petiole attached to the lower surface within the margin.

This species is very common and widely distributed in open places and second-growth forests throughout the Philippines.

Family SAPOTACEAE

Genus ACHRAS

ACHRAS SAPOTA L.   CHÍCO.

CHICLE GUM

Gum chicle, which is the principal substance used in the manufacture of chewing gum, is derived from the bark of this plant. In the Philippines, *Achras sapota* is extensively grown for its edible fruits known as chicos. No gum chicle is produced locally, although it would seem that it might be a profitable industry. The following short account of gum chicle is taken from the National Standard Dispensatory.[†]

Somewhat like Gutta-percha in its general nature is Chicle, or Gum

---

[*] Heyne, K., De Nuttige Planten van Nederlandsch-Indië, Volume 3 (1916), page 86.

[†] National Standard Dispensatory (1905), page 751.

Chicle, now the principal substance used in the manufacture of chewing-gum, and derived from *Achras Sapota* L. (*Sapota Achras* Mill., the *Sabodilla, Sapotilla, White sapota, Naseberry,* or *Ya,* of tropical America, where this tree supplies one of the most important edible fruits. Although the substance is collected in many parts of Mexico and Central America, the principal sources of supply are in Yucatan. The milk-juice is obtained from incisions made in the bark, performed with great care and by experienced persons. Tapping may occur once in 3 years without great danger to the life of the tree. The raw milk is boiled and then allowed to harden in brick-shaped moulds. If carefully prepared, it usually turns out of a white or whitish color, though that of some trees is said to turn out red in any case, a result which will also occur if the ordinary milk be overcooked. If undercooked, it retains a large percentage of water, proportionately reducing its value. Various devices for adulterating substances of this class are resorted to. Chicle gum of good quality is whitish, of firm, tenacious, somewhat elastic consistency, yet may be crumbled between the fingers; somewhat aromatic and nearly tasteless. It becomes plastic on chewing. Examined by Prochozka and Endemann, 75 per cent was found to be a resin, 9 per cent calcium oxalate (with traces of magnesium sulphate).

Concerning gum chicle, Hyde * states that:

* * * The best grades are nearly white and clean, but, if overheated, a red gum is produced. Consists of an oxidized hydrocarbon, closely related to caoutchouc. Softens in the mouth, and is tasteless but aromatic when heated. Sp. gr. 1.05. Soluble in chloroform, carbon tetrachloride, benzine, and somewhat in alcohol.

Uses.—Transmission belts, dental surgery, substitute for gutta percha, and more especially for chewing-gum.

According to Rogers,† the trees yield about six to eight pounds of gum. Most of the chicle imported into the United States is used in making chewing gum. For this purpose, washed and dried chicle is mixed with flavoring materials and fragrant oils.

Dannerth ‡ gives detailed methods for analyzing the crude gum. An idea of its composition may be obtained from the following figures (Dannerth) showing the analysis of a sample from Yucatan:

	Per cent.
Aceton-soluble matter (resins)	40.00
Gutta (and carbohydrates)	17.40
Proteins	0.60
Sand and foreign matter	2.30
Water	35.00
Mineral matter (ash)	4.70

* Hyde, F. S., Solvents, oils, gums, waxes and allied substances (1913), page 41.

† Rogers, A., Industrial chemistry (1915), page 722.

‡ Dannerth, F., Journal of Industrial and Engineering Chemistry, Volume 9 (1917), page 679.

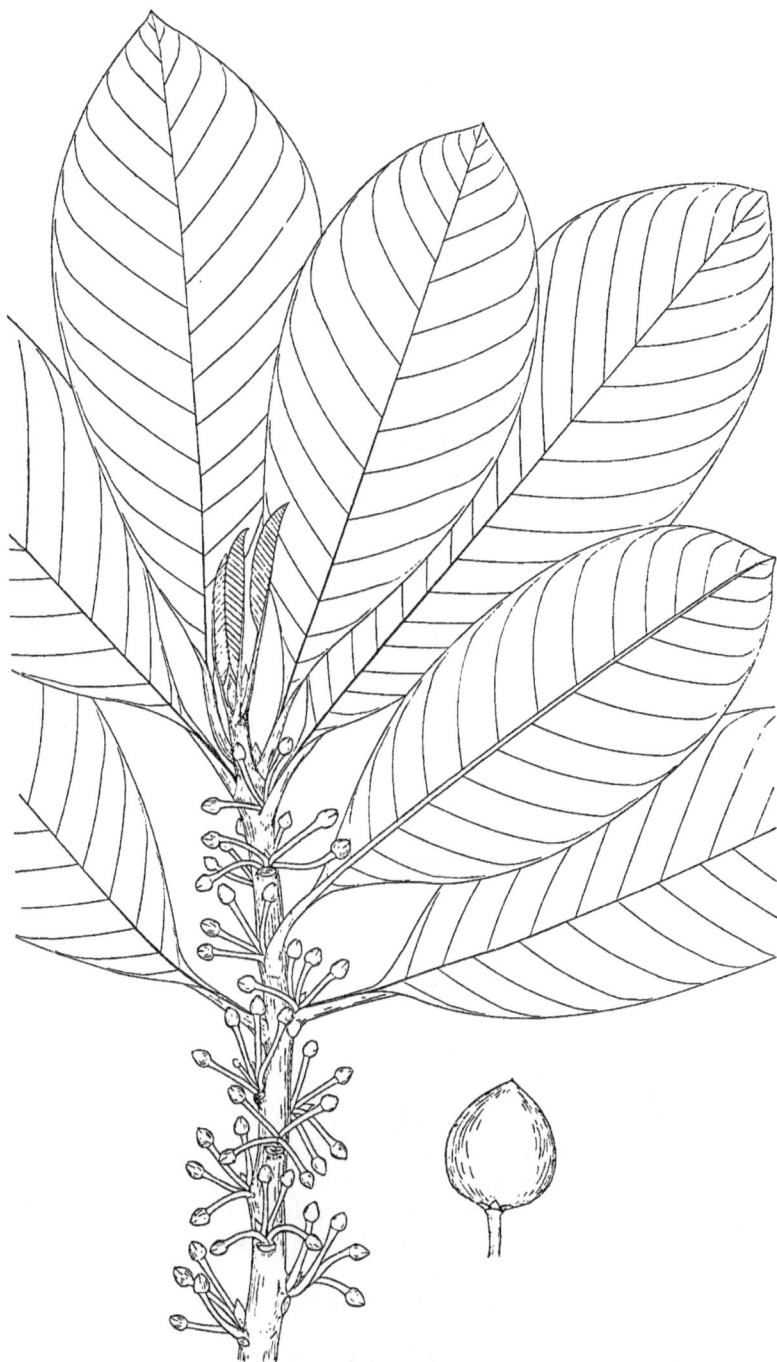

FIGURE 25. PALAQUIUM AHERNIANUM (KALIPÁYA), A SOURCE OF GUTTA-PERCHA.
X⅓.

Dannerth says that in 1916 approximately 7,347,000 pounds of chicle were imported into the United States. This is equivalent to about 30,000,000 pounds of chewing gum.

Genus PALAQUIUM

PALAQUIUM AHERNIANUM Merr. (Figs. 25–28).   KALIPÁYA.

Local names: *Kalapía, kalipáya* (Zamboanga); *salikút* (Surigao); *salukút* (Bukidnon).

GUTTA-PERCHA

A number of species of this genus produce gutta-percha. The Philippine species containing gutta-percha are numerous, but in most cases the grade is apparently too poor to make its collection profitable. The best known of the Philippine gutta-percha trees is *Palaqium ahernianum*. In the Philippines, commercial gutta-percha is apparently confined largely, if not entirely, to Mindanao and Tawi-Tawi. Here gutta-percha trees formerly existed in considerable numbers, but the method of collection has resulted in the destruction of the trees until, at the present time, the supply in accessible regions has been almost entirely depleted. Formerly considerable quantities of gutta-percha were exported from the Philippines, but now the amount exported is small. In Table 7, are given the exports for the years 1915 to 1918.

TABLE 7.—*Amount and value of gutta-percha exported from the Philippine Islands for the years 1915 to 1918.*

Year.	Amount.	Value.
	Kilo-grams.	*Pesos.*
1915	31,650	31,143
1916	29,962	22,898
1917	14,359	11,640
1918	2,334	2,007

Although the potential supply has been greatly depleted, the amount exported would increase considerably if the collectors received a higher price. At the present time gutta-percha is collected in a desultory manner and sold to Chinese merchants at a small price. It then passes through several hands and most of it finally reaches Singapore.

According to Sherman,* who made an extensive study of

---

* Sherman, Jr., P. L. The gutta-percha and rubber of the Philippine Islands. Bureau of Government Laboratories Publication No. 7 (1903), page 7.

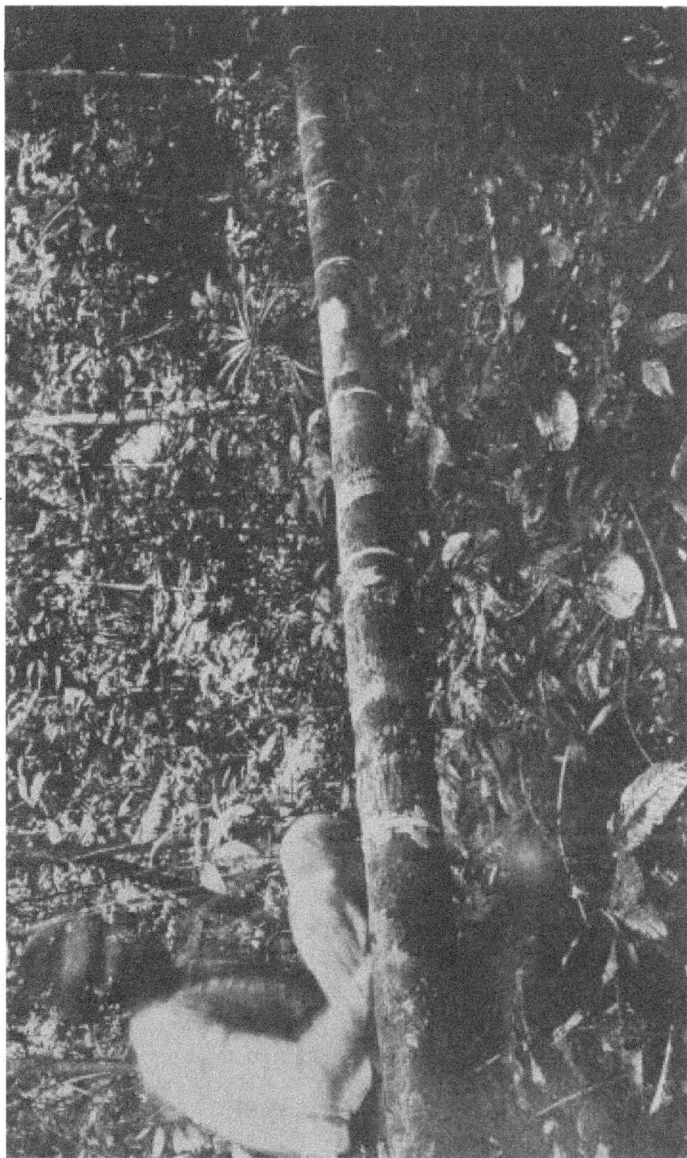

FIGURE 26. TAPPING A GUTTA-PERCHA TREE IN SUCH A MANNER THAT ALL THE MILK IS COLLECTED IN SHELLS BENEATH AND NONE LOST. DONE BY MOROS IN TAWI-TAWI.

gutta-percha in the Philippines, the usual method of collection is as follows:

* * * The tree is first cut down and the larger branches at once lopped off, the collectors say to prevent the gutta-percha milk from flowing back into the small branches and leaves. As has been previously stated the milk or latex is contained in the layers of the bark and leaves, in small capillary tubes or ducts. . . To open these so as to permit the maximum amount of the milk to escape, the natives cut rings in the bark about two feet apart along the entire length of the trunk. The milk as it flows out is collected in gourds, coconut shells, large leaves, or in some districts in the chopped-up bark itself, which is left adhering to the tree for the purpose of acting as a sort of sponge. * * *. After one or two hours, when the milk has ceased to flow, the contents of the receptacles are united and boiled over a fire for the purpose of finishing the partial coagulation. The warm, soft mass is then worked with cold water until a considerable amount of the liquid is mechanically inclosed. To further increase the weight, chopped bark, stones, etc., are added and the whole mass worked into the required shape with most of the dirt on the inside.

Sherman characterizes this method as very wasteful, since the tree usually falls in such a way that it is not possible to ring the trunk on all sides. He says:

* * * As a general thing from one-third to one-half of it is inaccessible to the process of ringing, and all the milk within this portion is consequently lost. Even the larger limbs are not deemed worth ringing and consequently all the milk in them and in the leaves also goes to waste; to this must be added the considerable quantity spilled on the ground through carelessness and lack of enough receptacles for every cut or bruise from which the milk flows.

Furthermore, no matter how much cutting is done, all of the milk will not flow from the trunk. Sherman collected a measured quantity of bark, after no more gutta-percha could be collected by the method described above, and extracted all of the gutta-percha which it contained. From this he estimated that ten times more gutta-percha was left than collected. Perhaps an even greater disadvantage of the usual method of collection is that it destroys the trees and therefore reduces the potential supply. Concerning this point Sherman states:

It is fortunate that only the full-grown trees contain enough gutta percha to repay the work of felling, ringing, etc.; otherwise the complete extermination of the gutta-percha forest would only be a matter of a year or so. On the other hand the felling of all the trees old enough to bear seed works to the same end with a somewhat longer time limit.

Gutta-percha is cleaned by the Chinese merchants, who ship it to Singapore. The account of this process given below is taken from a report by W. I. Hutchinson, formerly of the Bureau of Forestry:

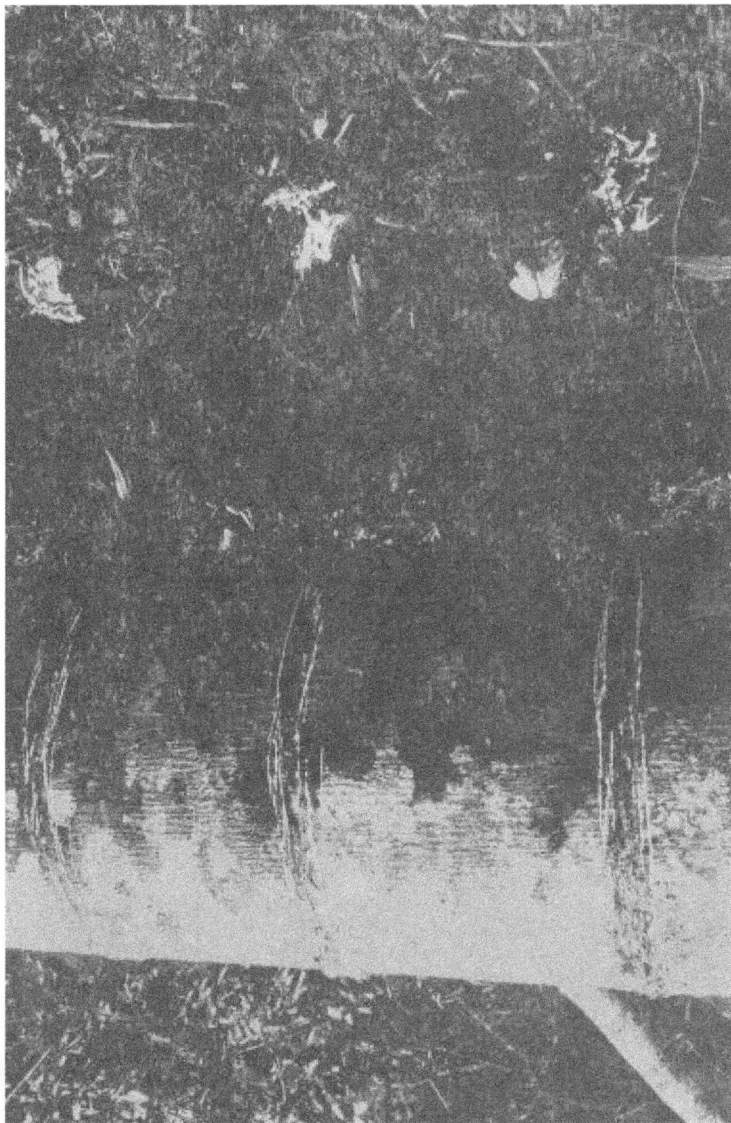

FIGURE 27. A GUTTA-PERCHA TREE TAPPED IN SUCH A MANNER THAT THE FLOWING MILK IS NOT ALL ABSORBED BY THE CHOPPED-UP BARK, BUT MUCH OF IT IS LOST ON THE GROUND BELOW. TUCURAN, DISTRICT OF ZAMBOANGA, MINDANAO.

The classification of gutta-percha depends largely on its flexibility, and freeness from bark and other forms of dirt. The first class product is almost pure white in color, and contains but a small amount of foreign matter. The second and third class gum has a pinkish tinge the amount of bark, stones, sticks, etc. varying from 20 per cent to 50 per cent or more.

First class or white gutta is rarely worked over, but the inferior grades are almost always subjected to a cleaning process before being shipped, on account of the low price that "dirty" gutta commands in the Singapore market.

The first step in the cleaning process is, to cut or tear the balls or rolls of gutta into small pieces. If the rolls are large they are often placed in hot water and allowed to soften slightly, in order to facilitate the separation of the sheets or strips.

As soon as a large amount of the product has been thus prepared, a fire is kindled under a stone oven, in the top of which a large caldron, three feet or more in diameter, has been sunk. This caldron is filled two-thirds full of water, the "scrap" gutta dumped in, and the whole mass allowed to boil until the gum becomes soft and stringy.

After boiling for a short time the bark contained in the "scrap" colors the water a deep blood-red-brown, and stains the softened gutta a pinkish tinge. Some of the Chinos add varying quantities of salt to the liquid, probably "to set" the color, although they one and all deny that this is the reason.

When the gutta is soft enough to be worked, it is dipped out with a bejuco sieve or a shovel, five or six quarts being placed in a heap upon a broad flat board. Over this steaming mass a sack is thrown, upon which a native, after dipping his feet in cold water, treads, thus causing the gum to spread out in a broad, flat sheet. If there is considerable dirt present it is usual to work over the mass with a large meat fork or a (paddle, shaking out as much of the bark, etc., as possible.

As soon as the forking process is finished, tramping is again resorted to, this time without the sack. When the gutta has again been worked into a sheet, water is thrown upon it, a native meanwhile brushing it vigorously with a stiff broom, and occasionally removing a large piece of dirt with his hands.

While the sheet is being turned over, the board on which it has been (resting is either brushed or washed clean.

Tramping is done altogether with the heels, the men maintaining their balance by holding to a rope stretched, some five feet above the ground, in front of the board.

After a time when the gutta becomes too hard to be dented by the heel, wooden mallets, or sticks similar to those used by the natives in hulling rice, are employed for beating.

At the completion of each tramping or beating operation, a sheet 2 ft. wide, 3 ft. or more in length, and 1 in. thick, is obtained, which is folded into as small a roll as possible, preparatory to the next tramping.

The cleaning operation being finished, the sheet is folded into an oblong mass, 12 in. long, 6 to 8 in. wide, and 5 in. thick, having a weight of from 8 to 12 pounds.

Three men, who receive a peso a day each, two working on the gutta and one carrying water, can clean three piculs per day.

Another method of cleaning gutta-percha is to boil it in

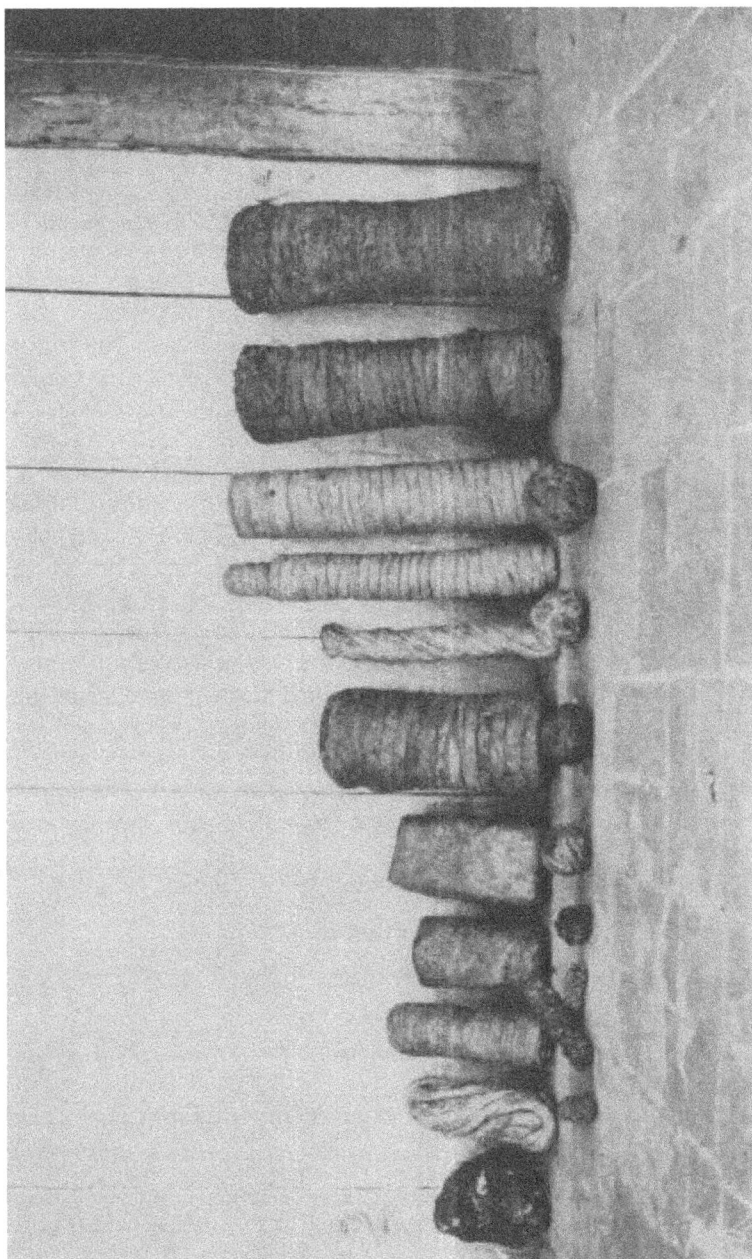

FIGURE 28. GUTTA-PERCHA AS IT REACHES THE MARKET.

water to which petroleum has been added. The petroleum is said to facilitate the removal of dirt and resin. After the first boiling the gutta-percha is ground and boiled again with water, the process being repeated several times. This method apparently results in a high-grade product.

Gutta-percha is now being grown successfully in plantations in a number of tropical countries, but not in the Philippines. According to Foxworthy: *

Successful extraction of gutta from the leaves is done by the Dutch and the cultural methods adopted in the plantation are devoted exclusively to leaf production. * * *

No great development of the gutta-percha industry in the Philippine Islands can be expected until the trees are grown in plantations.

The most important use of gutta-percha is for the insulation of submarine and underground electrical cables. It is also utilized considerably in the manufacture of surgical appliances, funnels, bottles, and other articles which come in frequent contact with acids. For these purposes it is valuable on account of the ease with which it can be sterilized and its resistance to acids. A familiar form is as the outer covering of golf balls.

Palaquium ahernianum is a tree reaching a height of about 40 meters and a diameter of 1.5 meters. The leaves are alternate, pointed at both ends, wider toward the tip than near the base, from 12 to 20 centimeters long, the lower surface velvety and with a rusty color. The flowers occur singly or in groups of two or three on wart-like growths on the stem. The fruits are one-seeded, somewhat rounded, and about 2.5 centimeters in diameter.

This species is apparently confined to Mindanao.

Genus PAYENA

PAYENA LEERII Kurz. (Fig. 29).

GUTTA-PERCHA

According to Heyne † this tree produces a very good grade of gutta-percha.

This species has been collected once in Mindanao and once in Tawi-Tawi.

---

* Foxworthy, F. W., Minor forest products and jungle produce. Government of British North Borneo, Department of Forestry Bulletin No. 1, Part II (1916), page 45.

† Heyne, K., De Nuttige Planten van Nederlandsch-Indië, Volume 4 (1917), page 12.

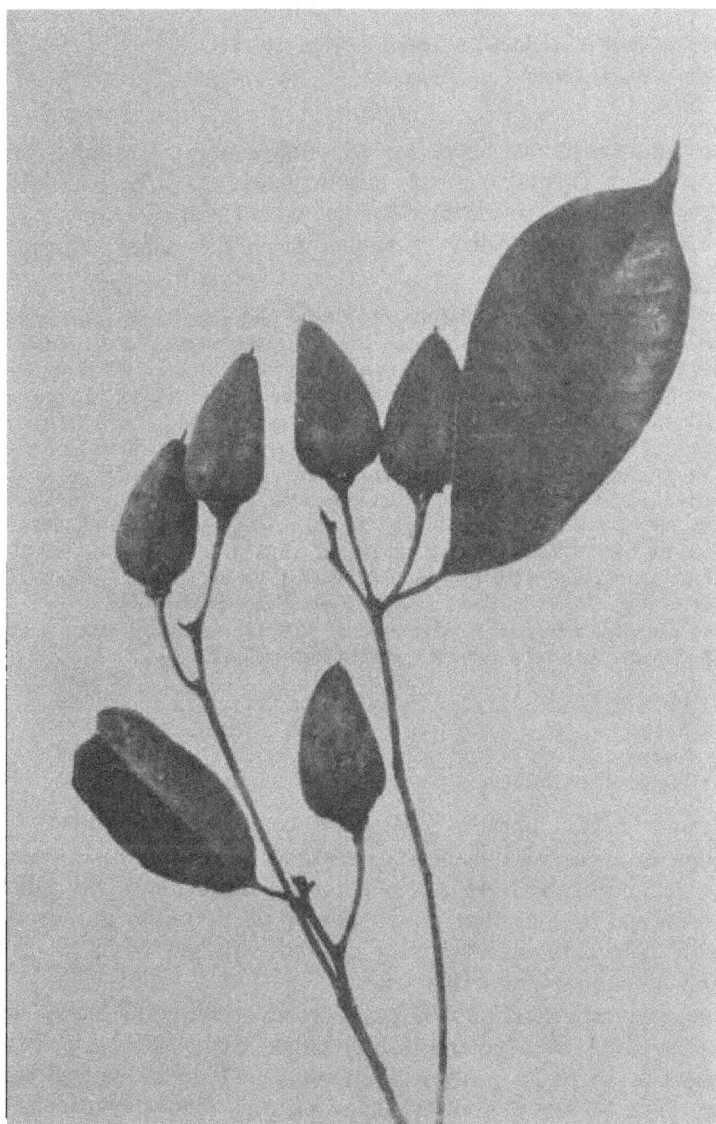

FIGURE 29. LEAVES AND FRUIT OF PAYENA LEERII, A SOURCE OF GUTTA-PERCHA.

168837——6

Family APOCYNACEAE

Genus CHONEMORPHA

CHONEMORPHA ELASTICA Merr. (Figs. 30, 31).   LISID.
Local names: *Goma, lisid* (Apayao).

RUBBER

In the Philippines there are a number of species of native plants which furnish rubber, but the only one known to yield rubber of a high grade is *Chonemorpha elastica.* Concerning the collection and quality of rubber from this plant, Sherman writes:*

The Philippine rubber collectors are Samal and Joloano Moros living in ' Tawi-Tawi and the adjacent coral islands. The method of coagulation used by them was undoubtedly learned from the Moros of North Borneo, who with the Dyaks collect much of the rubber in that island. It consists in first pulling the vine down to the ground so as to be better able to tap it along its entire length. The milk is caught in cocoanut shells or leaves, and coagulated by pouring into sea water. The coagulation is almost instantaneous, and when properly manipulated a large amount of water can be mechanically inclosed inside the large balls along with plenty of chopped-up bark. The resulting rubber, of which I secured many samples, is white, tough, and very elastic so long as it is kept in sea water. On exposure to the air it blackens and decomposition slowly sets in.

The chemical analysis of a sample of this rubber, after much of the dirt and water had been removed, resulted as follows:

	Per cent.
Dirt	3.76
Rubber	81.57
Resins	3.16
Water	11.51

Formerly this species existed in considerable numbers in Basilan and Tawi-Tawi, but the method of collection described above has naturally lessened the potential supply, and will reduce it to such an extent that it will not be profitable to gather the rubber. No extensive industry can be expected from the collection of rubber from this vine.

Chonemorpha elastica is a large, woody vine. The leaves are opposite, thin, rounded or slightly pointed at the base, pointed at the tip, 15 to 20 centimeters long, and 8 to 15 centimeters wide. The flowers are white, fragrant, and about 3 centimeters wide.

This species has been reported from Cagayan, Apayao, Benguet, Cavite, Mindanao, Basilan, and Tawi-Tawi.

---

* Sherman, Jr., P. L. The gutta-percha and rubber of the Philippine ' Islands. Bureau of Government Laboratories Publication No. 7 (1903), page 39.

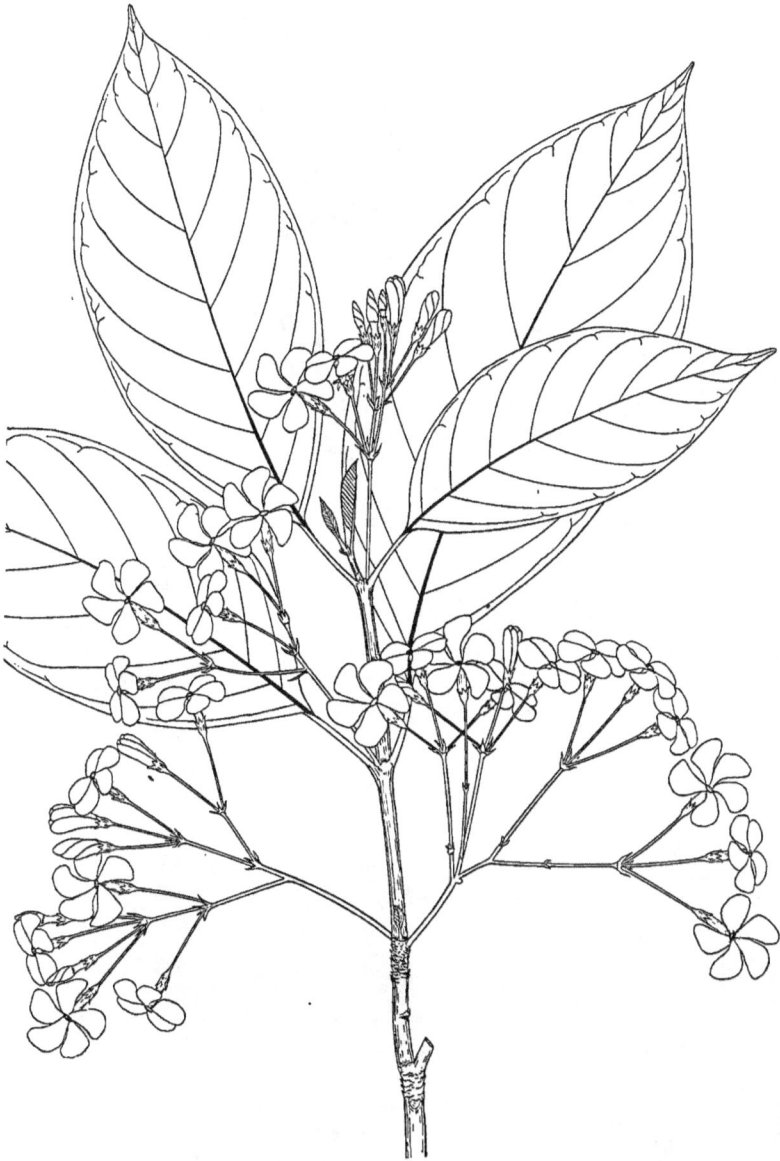

FIGURE 30. CHONEMORPHA ELASTICA (LISID), A RUBBER VINE. ×⅓.

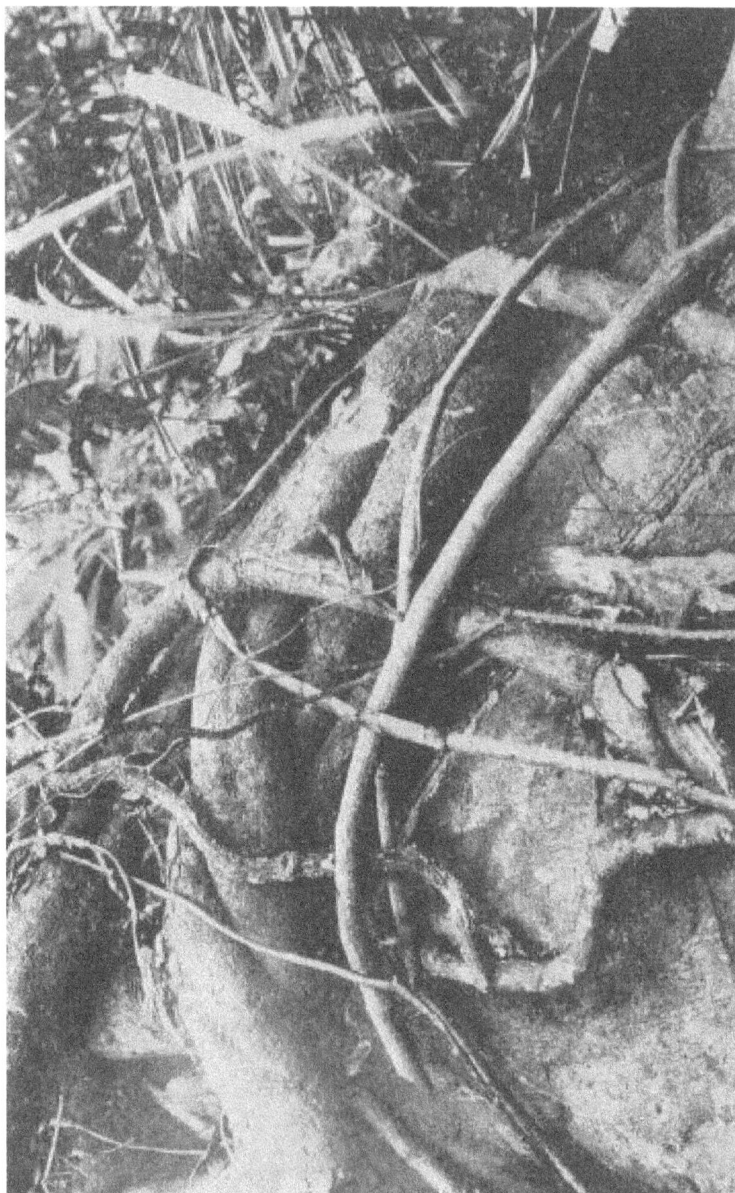

FIGURE 31. CHONEMORPHA ELASTICA (A RUBBER VINE) IN THE FOREST.

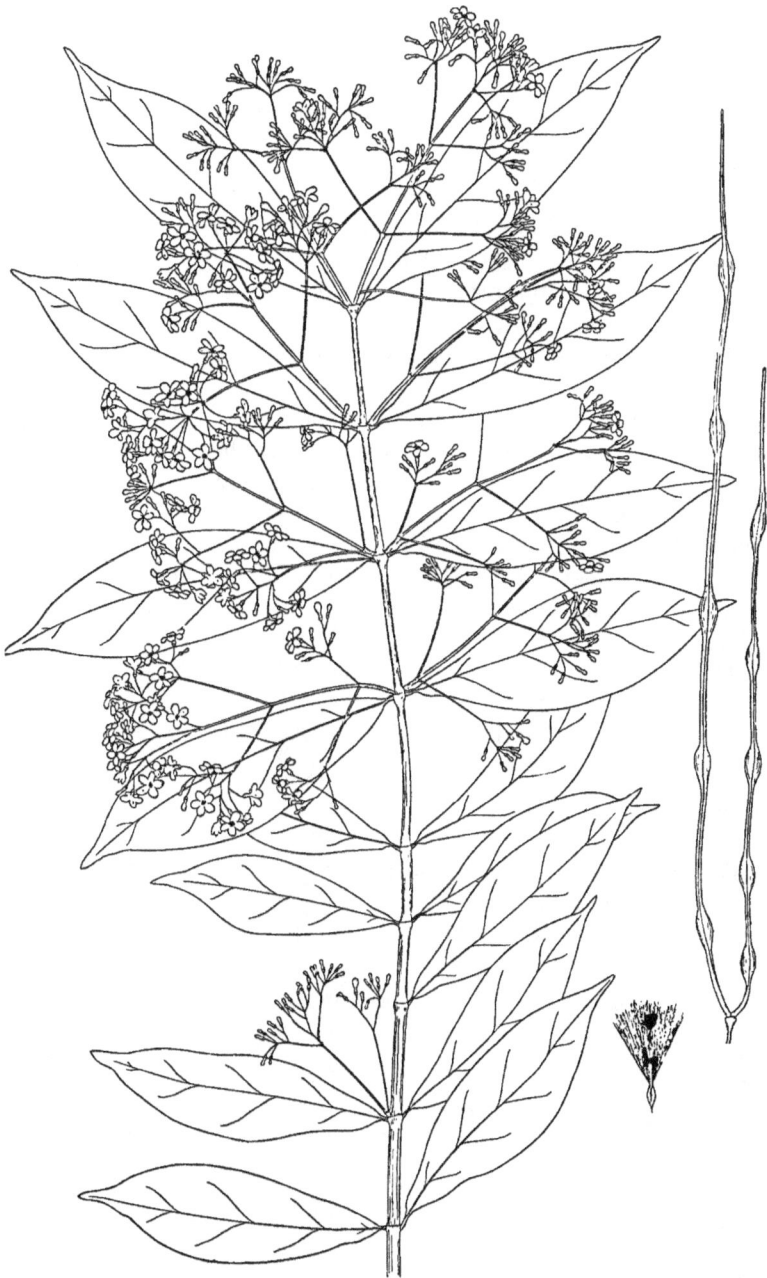

FIGURE 32. PARAMERIA PHILIPPINENSIS, (DUGTUNG-AHAS) A RUBBER VINE. X½.

Genus **PARAMERIA**

PARAMERIA PHILIPPINENSIS Radlk. (Figs. 32, 33). DUGTUNG-ÁHAS.
Local names: *Dugtung-áhas* (Rizal); *ikdíng ñga púrau* (Igorot); *inggíu na putí* (Bataan); *karkarsáng* (Benguet); *kuni na putí* (Pampanga); *lupí-it* (Ilocos Sur); *parugtong-áhas* (Bulacan, Zambales, Rizal); *partaán* (Ilocos Sur); *pulang-pulang* (Zambales); *sada* (Benguet); *taguláuai* (Rizal).

RUBBER

This species yields rubber which is seemingly of rather poor grade. It has never been collected to any great extent. Locally the vine is apparently better known as a snake medicine than as a rubber plant.

The bark of this species is also used for making rope and for tying rice bundles.

Parameria philippinensis is a woody vine. The leaves are from 7 to 10 centimeters in length, somewhat oval in outline, and pointed at both ends. The flowers are fairly small, white, and occur in clusters. The fruits are very long and slender; the parts between the seeds are very narrow. The seeds are about a centimeter in length, sharply pointed at one end, and at the other end crowned with numerous white hairs about 2.5 centimeters long.

This species is common and is widely distributed in the Philippines.

Family BORRAGINACEAE

Genus **CORDIA**

CORDIA MYXA L.   ANÓNANG.

ANÓNANG GUM

A description of this species and its local names are given in the bulletin on fibers.

Locally, a paste is prepared from the fruits.

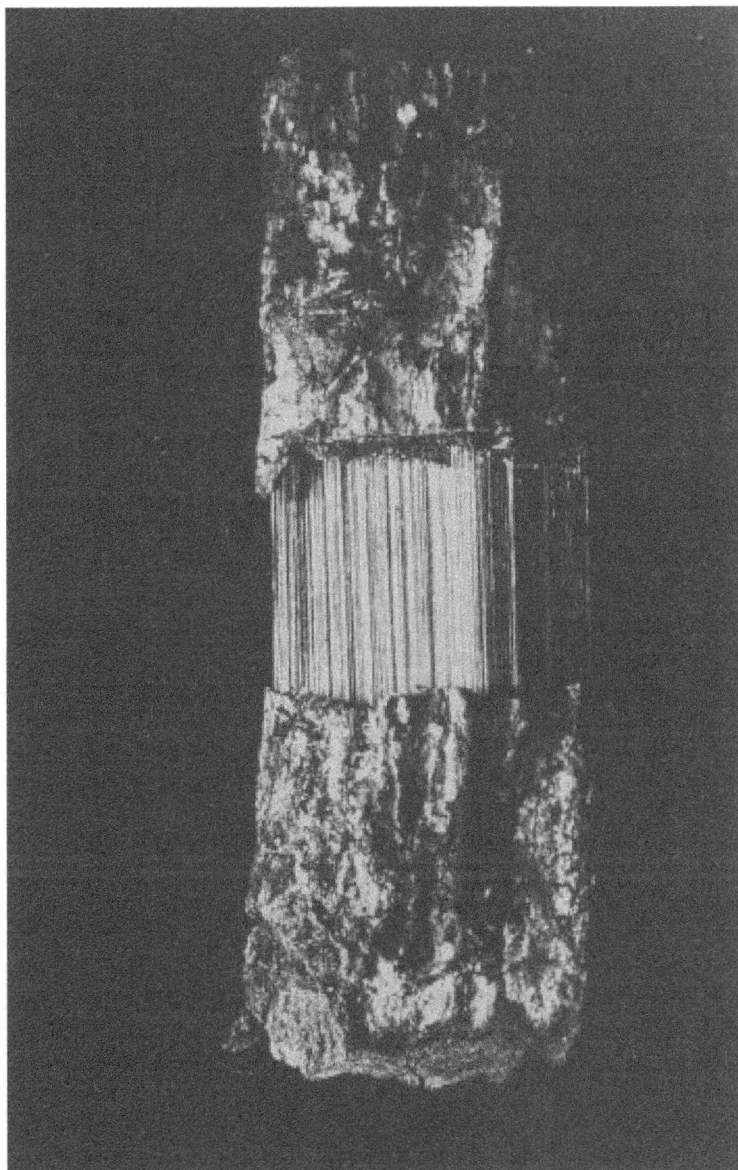

FIGURE 33. A PIECE OF DRY BARK FROM PARAMERIA PHILIPPINENSIS, BROKEN AND PULLED APART, SHOWING THE RUBBER.

SEED OILS

Vegetable oils are found naturally in the seeds of plants, and in many species the oil accumulates in considerable quantities. Many of these seed oils are edible, while others are useful for their medicinal properties or for the manufacture of paints, soaps, candles, or other practical purposes. In general, to obtain these oils, the seeds are first shelled. Although the oil may be obtained usually from the shelled seeds by extraction with organic solvents such as ether, the more general method is to subject the dried, shelled seeds to pressure. This process expels the oil, leaving a dried, crushed meal known as oil cake. The cake may be used for various purposes, depending upon its composition. If it does not contain injurious substances, it may be utilized for cattle food. Sometimes the oil cake is also employed as fertilizer or fuel. The expelled oil is filtered and, if necessary, subjected to further methods of refinement.

Edible oils usually contain both solid and liquid fats. Since fat is generally recognized as an indispensable constituent of human food, these edible oils are consequently substances of considerable importance. The fatty oils are sometimes called fixed oils, because when a drop of one of these oils is placed on wood it forms a rather permanent spot which does not evaporate readily on exposure to the air.

Fats (glycerides) consist essentially of glycerol (glycerin) combined with certain fatty acids such as oleic, palmitic, and stearic. The fats are usually insoluble in water, but dissolve readily in organic solvents. When boiled with an alkali solution they are decomposed (saponified) and converted into the alkali salts (soaps) of the fatty acids present, and glycerol. When fats, or edible oils containing fats, are exposed to light and air for a considerable length of time, they gradually decompose, forming free acids and other products, which have an unpleasant taste and odor. Oil which has been decomposed in this manner is said to be rancid. When decomposition has begun, the presence of micro-organisms appears to hasten these chemical changes. If the dried seeds are prepared properly and the oil obtained from them properly preserved, this decomposition can be hindered greatly and in some cases prac-

88

tically prevented. This is especially true of coconut oil, as Walker * has shown. Edible oils which are rancid and have a high acidity are not suited for edible purposes. Such oils are used largely for soap making. Since edible oils command a much higher price than soap oils, it is evident that when edible oils are allowed to become rancid the oil producer suffers considerable loss.

Investigation has shown that each particular oil has certain definite physical and chemical constants such as specific gravity, refractive index, saponification value, iodine value, etc. For a given oil, the exact value of these constants would naturally be affected by the purity of a particular sample and perhaps other factors. The results obtained by determining these various constants (oil analysis) are very useful in ascertaining the purity of a particular sample of a known oil or in endeavoring to identify an unknown one.

Lewkowitsch,[†] Allen,[‡] Mitchell,[§] Woodman,[‖] and various other authorities give explicit directions for making oil analyses and explain how the results may be interpreted.

In recent years the demand for edible oils has been steadily increasing. As a result of this tendency, efforts have been made to convert oils formerly used for making soaps and candles into edible oils, which are considerably more valuable. For this purpose the method which has proved most successful is known as hydrogenation. This process consists in converting fatty oils, which are liquid at ordinary temperatures, into hard, solid fats. The liquid fats consist largely of olein, which is a combination of oleic acid and glycerol (oleic glyceride); solid fats consist largely of stearin, a combination of stearic acid and glycerol (stearic glyceride). The glycerides comprising the hard portion of an oil contain more hydrogen than those forming the soft portion. It is possible, then, to harden the soft portion by merely adding a small amount of hydrogen, which is a well-known chemical gas. The hydrogenation process has been used successfully for preparing oils suitable for the soap and candle industries and also for making edible oils. Not only are soft oils hardened by hydrogenation, but certain of their oil constants

---

* Walker, H. S. The keeping qualities and the causes of rancidity in coconut oil. Philippine Journal of Science, Section A, Volume 1 (1906), page 117.

† Lewkowitsch, J. Oils, fats, and waxes. (1915), Volume 1.

‡ Allen, Commercial organic analysis. (1910), Volume 2.

§ Mitchell, C. A. Edible oils and fats, (1918).

‖ Woodman, A. G. Food analysis, (1915).

are changed considerably. This is especially true of the iodine value, which is decreased greatly, and of the specific gravity, which is increased.

The question of the edibility of hydrogenated oils has been discussed to some extent in chemical literature.*

It seems to be generally accepted by those who have investigated the matter carefully that the hydrogenated oils have as desirable a degree of edibility as the oils from which they are derived. It is even claimed that by destroying traces of certain unsaturated bodies thought to be slightly toxic in nature, hydrogenation renders the oil better adapted for human consumption.

Concerning the hydrogenation of oils, Thompson † states:

The combined capacity of the hydrogenating plants of Europe is esti- mated for 1914 at 250,000 tons (1,375,000 barrels), which is two or three times as much as has ever been treated. These plants are in England, Norway, Germany, and France, and are engaged at present chiefly on fats for soap and candles. They are hardening linseed, whale, soya-bean, and cottonseed oils.

The great increase in the demand for margarin in Europe, for com- pound lard in the United States, and for hard soap all over the civilized world has resulted in closely crowding the supply of natural hard fats, while liquid oils are relatively abundant. A few years ago strictly edible liquid oils seemed to be growing scarcer, but the new scheme of deodoriza- tion began to relieve this shortage by lifting the so-called soap oils into the edible class. The same process was applied to copra and palm-kernel oils, and finally caused a scarcity of soap greases. Hydrogenation now promises a further readjustment of conditions by permitting the transfer at will of any oil from the liquid to the solid class, and it will bring into use some relatively rare oils, and encourage the production of still others.

In producing oils intended for edible purposes, it is obvious that the highest grade of purity is desirable, to obtain which, the raw materials, such as seeds or fruits, should be selected carefully, and worked up rapidly, in as fresh a condition as possible. Special care should be observed to avoid the presence of considerable quantities of free fatty acids, since these sub- stances tend to decompose the oils and cause rancidity.

Seed oils which contain toxic substances are naturally unsuited for edible purposes. Such oils frequently have properties which make them especially valuable for various other purposes, such as the manufacture of medicinal preparations, paints, varnishes, etc. Certain seed oils, for instance, have unusual drying prop- erties which make them useful as paint oils. Linseed oil, which

---

* Ellis, C. The hydrogenation of oils (1919), page 323.

† Thompson, E. W. Cottonseed products and their competitors in northern Europe. Department of Commerce, Special Agents Series No. 89. Part II, Edible oils, 1914, page 26.

has the property of absorbing oxygen from the air and forming a dry, hard coating, is the most important of the drying oils and is employed extensively in making paints and varnishes. Philippine lumbang oil is also an excellent drying oil.

Andés * gives the composition of numerous oil cakes and discusses the practical application of these materials as cattle foods or fertilizers.

FAMILY PALMAE

Genus COCOS

COCOS NUCIFERA L. (Figs. 34–37).   COCONUT PALM.

COCONUT OIL

Coconut oil, which is derived from the fleshy kernels of *Cocos nucifera,* is far more important in the commerce of the Philippines than all other oils combined. An adequate discussion of an agricultural subject such as this would require so much space as to be out of place in a publication dealing primarily with forest products. As explained in the preface, there are very few important oils derived from cultivated plants in the Philippines, and so it has seemed advisable to include a short account of these in the present bulletin.

High-grade coconut oil is edible and is employed largely in making edible fats and artificial butter (margarine or oleomargarine). The lower and cheaper grades, which usually contain a considerable proportion of free fatty acids, are not suitable for food and are used principally for making soaps and candles. Coconut oil is also used in cooking, as an illuminant, and for various other purposes, such as the preparation of lotions, salves, and hair cosmetics. The uses of the different products of the coconut palm have been discussed by Miller † and by Brown and Merrill.‡

The usual method of obtaining coconut oil is essentially as follows: The husks are first removed from the nuts, after which they are split by a large knife and the milk poured off. The split nuts are next dried in the sun, or by artificial heat, after which the dried meat or copra is easily removed from the shells. The copra is then ground in a mill, heated, and subjected to pressure. The oil cake which remains after the first expression

---

* Andés, L. E., and Stocks, H. B., Vegetable fats and oils, (1917), page 323.

† Miller, H. H., Commercial geography, the materials of commerce for the Philippines, (1911).

‡ Brown, Wm. H., and Merrill, E. D., Philippine palms and palm products. Bureau of Forestry Bulletin No. 18 (1919).

still contains a considerable quantity of oil. In some mills this cake is subjected to a second expression by means of hydraulic presses after which it contains only a slight percentage of oil. The coconut oil obtained is filtered and stored in large tanks, ready for domestic use or export. The oil cake, which remains after the oil has been expressed, is used as cattle food or, sometimes, as fertilizer or fuel.

In recent years the demand and prices for animal fats, such as lard and butter, have been steadily growing and it seems that there will probably be a permanent shortage of animal fats. This has led to a greatly increased use of vegetable fats by European and American makers of artificial butter, resulting in an unusual demand for these vegetable products. Coconut oil, which was formerly utilized largely in making soaps and candles, is the most popular ingredient of artificial butter.

* * * Marseilles, which is the most important soap-manufacturing city in Europe, requires annually something like 120,000 tons of fat for this industry. Heretofore 40 per cent of this has been coconut oil. But in recent years, out of the total production of 85,000 tons of copra oil in Marseilles, about 50,000 tons are sold direct as an edible fat, and 10,000 tons are exported to the Netherlands and elsewhere for mixing with cottonseed oil, peanut oil, and other soft fats to make oleomargarin; this leaves but 25,000 tons for the soap trade there, when the normal supply from this source has been 48,000 tons.*

As a result of the increased demand for coconut oil, new coconut plantations are being developed, and it is said that some of the margarine manufacturers have acquired plantations and oil mills, so that they may control their own raw product. These trade conditions in vegetable fats have naturally affected the Philippines, which is one of the largest coconut-producing countries in the world.

Formerly, a large proportion of Philippine coconuts were converted into copra, which was shipped to the United States and European countries where the oil was expressed. When copra is allowed to stand for a considerable length of time before shipment it tends to deteriorate, causing a loss in the quality and quantity of the oil. Obviously, in so far as this deterioration is concerned, it is more economical to produce the oil in the countries where the coconuts are grown. This would logically reduce the bulk of the shipments and avoid possible losses due to spoiling. The recent shortage of shipping space naturally

---

* Brill, H. C. and Agcaoili, F., Philippine oil-bearing seeds and their properties: II. Philippine Journal of Science, Section A, Volume 10 (1915), page 106.

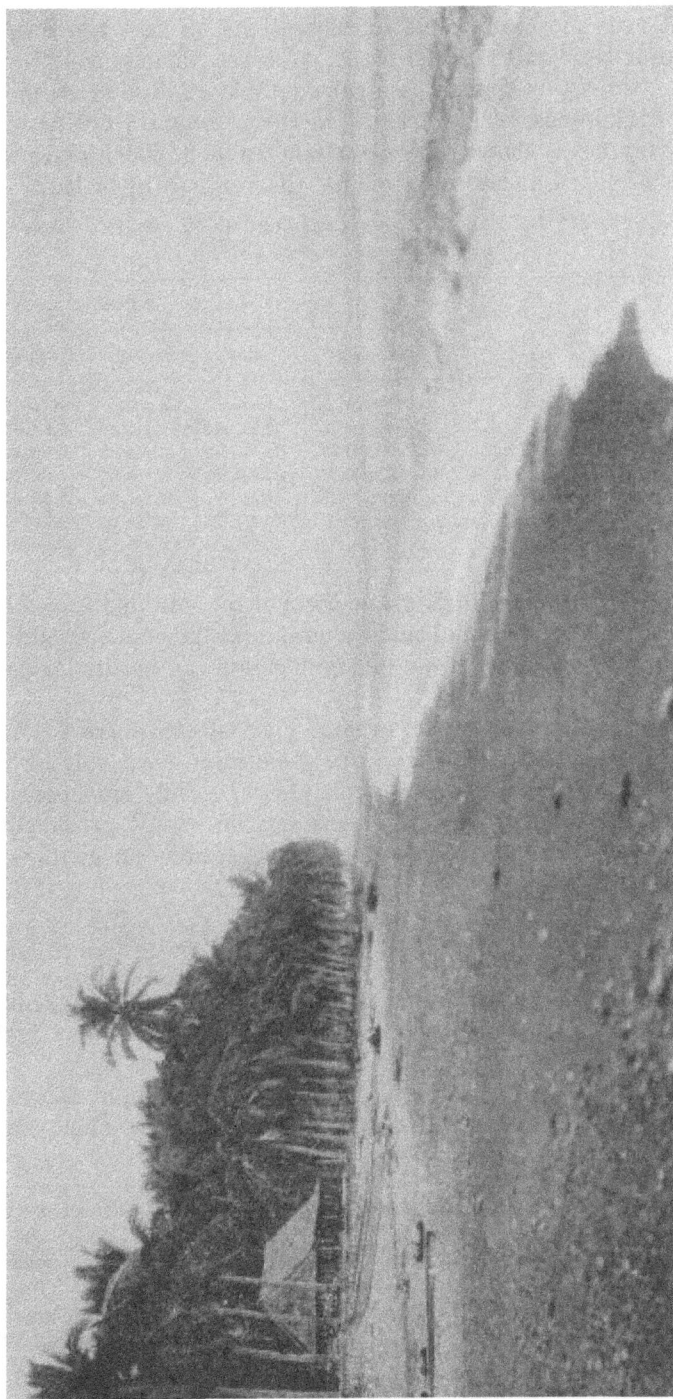

FIGURE 34. COCONUT PALMS GROWING ON THE BEACH AT SAN RAMON, MINDANAO.

made it even more advisable to express the oil near the source of coconut production. The result of these various conditions has been the establishment of a considerable number of oil mills in the Philippines. The increase in the coconut-oil business in the Philippines is shown very clearly in Table 8, which gives the exports of copra and coconut oil for the years 1913 to 1918.

TABLE 8.—*Amount and value of copra and coconut oil exported from the Philippines from 1913 to 1918.*

Year.	Copra.		Coconut oil.	
	Amount.	Value.	Amount.	Value.
	Kilograms.	*Pesos.*	*Kilograms.*	*Pesos.*
1913	82,219,363	19,091,448	5,010,429	2,292,678
1914	87,344,695	15,960,540	11,943,329	5,238,366
1915	139,092,902	22,223,109	13,464,169	5,641,003
1916	72,277,164	14,231,941	16,091,169	7,851,469
1917	92,180,326	16,654,301	45,198,415	22,818,294
1918	55,061,736	10,377,029	115,280,847	63,328,317

In order to produce high-grade coconut oil, suitable for edible purposes, only ripe nuts should be used, and the copra should be dried properly. These two important points can hardly be over-emphasized.

Ripe coconuts give a much greater yield of copra and coconut oil than green nuts. Coconuts are sometimes, carelessly or intentionally, cut from the tree before they are fully ripe, causing considerable financial loss. Concerning the use of green nuts, Walker,† who has made extensive investigations on copra and coconut oil, states:

* * * The percentage of anhydrous copra in the meat of the green fruit is 33.7; it rises to 50.1 in that of the "fairly ripe" nuts and increases to 53.3 in those marked "dead ripe." * * * Only thoroughly ripe nuts (the husks of which have begun to turn brown) should be used, and it is often advisable to allow the latter to stand in a dry place for a few weeks before they are opened. * * *

Walker also says that there appears to be a slight increase in the proportion of meat, copra, and oil in nuts which have been stored, up to a maximum of three months after cutting;

---

† Walker, H. S., The coconut and its relation to the production of coconut oil. Philippine Journal of Science, Volume 1 (1906), page 71.

Walker, H. S., The keeping qualities and causes of rancidity in coconut oil. Philippine Journal of Science, Volume 1 (1906), page 140.

Walker, H. S., Notes on the sprouting coconut, on copra, and on coconut oil. Philippine Journal of Science, Section A, Volume 3 (1908), page 126.

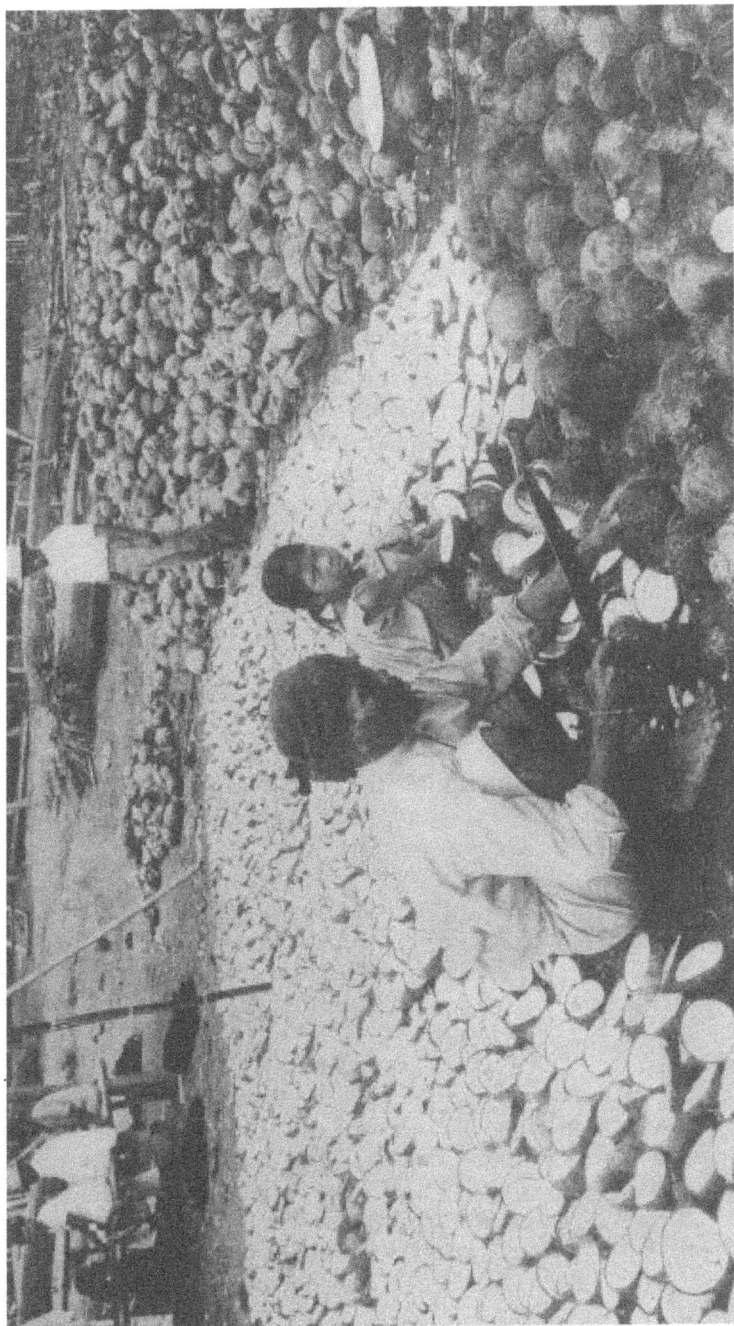

FIGURE 35. OPENING COCONUTS FOR DRYING AT PAGSANJAN, LAGUNA.

and that beyond this period, which coincides with the time that the sprout makes its appearance, there is a decided decrease in the above constituents.

The quality and value of coconut oil depend largely upon the condition of the copra at the time of milling. Copra which has not been sufficiently dried becomes moldy. The molds tend to decompose, or hydrolyze the fats in the copra, with the result that the oil, after expression, contains free, fatty acids, becomes rancid quickly, and acquires a bad odor. Walker made a large number of experiments to determine the conditions which induce this deterioration and the methods by which it could be prevented. He found that, ordinarily, commercial copra contained from 9 to 12 per cent of moisture and that this amount was very favorable for the growth of molds. Most of the free acids and the accompanying bad odor and taste which are present in coconut oil are produced in the copra itself. Walker found that no organisms grew, and that there was no change of acidity, in a sample of copra containing 4.7 per cent of moisture. The remedy is to dry the copra until it contains no more than 5 per cent of moisture, which prevents the growth of mold; and to express the oil as soon as possible, thereby avoiding long storage in a warm, moist atmosphere. He says that the copra should be fresh and be prepared under the best possible conditions of drying, and that the oil should be thoroughly dried and filtered until absolutely clear. Under these conditions it should be capable of shipment or storage without noticeable deterioration. He believed, contrary to many statements, that the keeping qualities of coconut oil prepared in a pure state were superior to those of most other vegetable fats and oils. When sufficient sugars and albuminoids are left in the oil, if, in other words, it is not properly filtered, molds which have been pressed out with the oil or, in the case of hot-pressed oil, which enter the freshly prepared oil, cause a rapid splitting of the fat and an increase in acidity.

Brill, Parker, and Yates * confirmed Walker's conclusions, that the deterioration of copra is due largely to molds and not to bacteria, since a moisture content sufficiently high to favor bacterial growth is not found ordinarily in copra and, moreover, bacteria cause scarcely any loss even under conditions most favorable for their growth. These writers found four molds occurring upon coconut meat and moldy copra. The spore masses of the four molds differ considerably in color and are

---

* Brill, H. C., Parker, H. O., and Yates, H. S., Copra and coconut oil. Philippine Journal of Science, Section A, Volume 12 (1917), page 55.

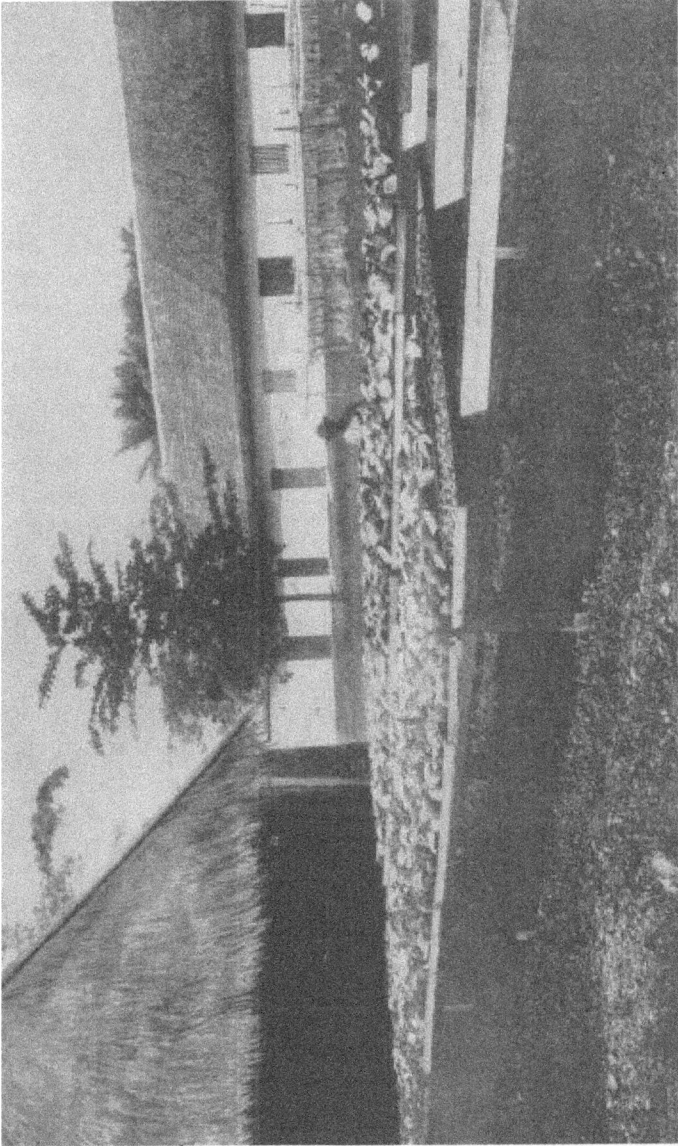

FIGURE 36. SUN-DRYING COCONUTS, SHOWING THE NUTS ON THE TRAYS READY TO BE PUSHED UNDER THE SHELTER.

168837——7

easily distinguished without the aid of a microscope. These
molds are given below in the order of their moisture require-
ments; the first one needing the most moisture for growth and
the last one the least.

White mold, *Rhizopus* sp. This mold occurs only on fresh
meat in a practically saturated atmosphere. It forms loose
masses of white threads, with many black sporangia.

Black mold, *Aspergillus niger*, Van Teigh. A mold which
occurs in copra with a relatively high moisture content and
produces black spore bodies, giving the mold a black color.

Brown or yellow mold, *Aspergillus flavus*, Link. This species
is the most common one on moldy copra. The spore masses,
which are at first greenish yellow, gradually become brown.

Green mold, *Penicillium glaucum* Link. This mold produces
green spores, and occurs commonly on copra, especially if it
contains a low percentage of moisture. It causes very little
loss of oil.

Experiments showed that the brown mold, which occurs on
copra having a small moisture content, under ordinary conditions caused much more damage than the others. Under conditions favorable for its growth, this mold caused in one month
a loss of 30 to 40 per cent of the total oil. The oil also contained a considerable amount of free fatty acids and was of
poor quality.

According to Brill, Parker, and Yates, copra which has been
dried to a moisture content of about 6 per cent does not absorb
water and become moldy unless stored in a saturated atmosphere for prolonged periods of time.

The Bureau of Science in Manila frequently receives for analysis samples from the various coconut-oil mills in the Philippines.
Reports on these analyses made during the latter part of the
year 1919 have been compiled by the Division of Organic Chemistry. Their results show that Philippine coconut oil has the
following average specific gravity (degrees centigrade) $\frac{30°}{4°} =$
0.91461. The fatty acids, calculated as oleic acid, usually average 4 to 5 per cent. The results of a large number of analyses
of copra and copra cake are given in Table 9. These figures,
based upon general factory conditions throughout the whole archipelago, represent percentages as nearly correct as can be
obtained.

The figures given in Table 9 are based upon fresh hydraulic
and expeller cake, and not on cake stored for several months.
The latter would show an exceedingly high, free fatty acid con-

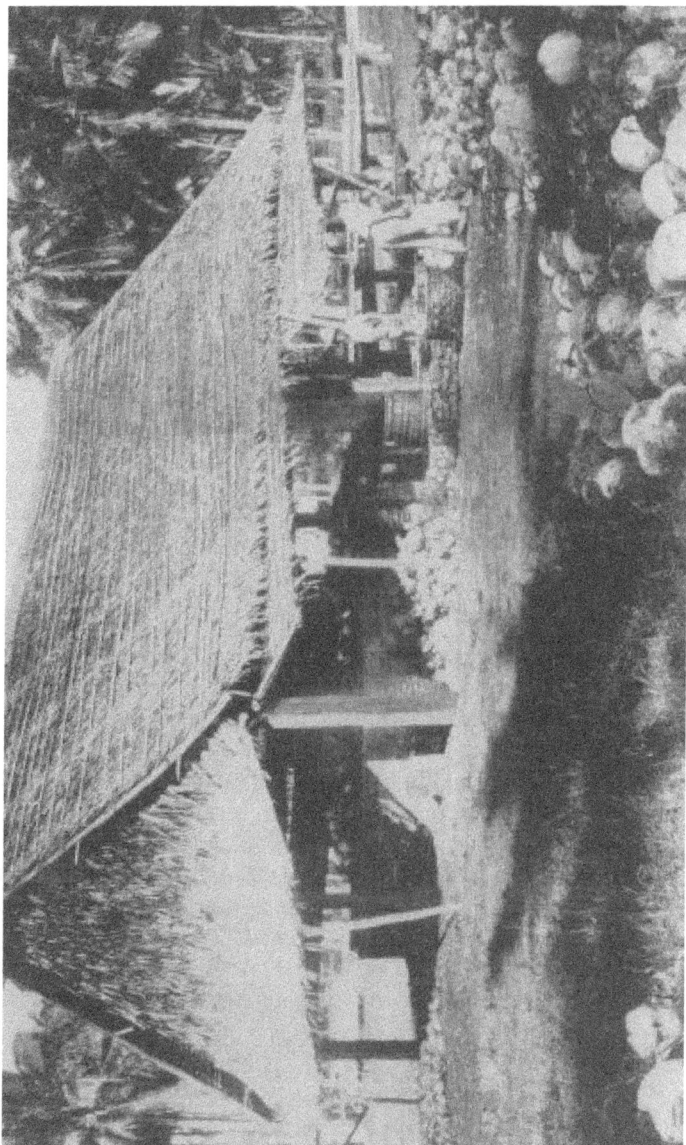

FIGURE 37. KILN USED FOR DRYING COCONUTS.

tent. In compiling these results, unusual analyses representing small quantities of either exceedingly good or poor copra have not been included. These exceptional samples have· shown a percentage of oil as high as 71, or as low as 57.5.

TABLE 9.—*Analysis of copra and copra cake.*

[Compiled by Division of Organic Chemistry, Bureau of Science.]

Constants.	Copra. Percentage.			Copra cake. Percentage.					
	Maximum.	Minimum.	Average.	Maximum.		Minimum.		Average.	
				Ex-peller.	Hy-draulic.	Ex-peller.	Hy-draulic.	Ex-peller.	Hy-draulic.
Oil	67.4	62	65.5	15.5	6.0	10.5	4.0	12.5	5.0
Ash				5.97		5.78		5.90	
Crude fiber				10.92		7.85		9.5	
Protein				21.44		16.8		19.9	
Moisture	7.0	4.5	5.5	9.2		4.0		5.38	
Free fatty acids calculated as oleic acid	6.2	3.0	4.8	12.0		4.0		7.2	

Coconut oil in temperate climates, at ordinary temperatures, is a solid fat, but in tropical countries it is usually a thick liquid. The high-grade oil is nearly colorless, has a bland taste, and the peculiar odor of coconuts. It consists largely of the glycerol esters of lauric and myristic acids and contains also a number of other fats which are the glycerol esters of still other fatty acids, such as caproic, capryllic, capric, and oleic. The exact composition of coconut oil is somewhat uncertain.

The physical and chemical constants of the oil obtained from different localities are given by various authorities as follows:

Specific gravity $\begin{cases} 15.5° \\ 18° \end{cases}$	0.9259
	0.9250
Solidifying point	15.7–23
Melting point	23–25
Saponification value	255–260
Iodine value	8–9.5
Reichert value	3.5–3.7
Reichert-Meissl value	6.7–7.5
Hehner value	88.6–90.5
Polenske value	16.8
Refractive index, 60°	1.441
Butyro refractometer 15.5°	49.1
Viscosity (seconds at 140°F.)	63.9–64.7

Genus ELAEIS

ELAEIS GUINEENSIS Jacq.   Oil Palm.

PALM OIL

This species yields two kinds of oil, known as palm oil and palm-kernel oil. Palm oil is obtained from the fleshy part of the fruit while the palm-kernel oil is expressed from the kernels. The uses of palm-kernel oil, for edible and technical purposes, are increasing considerably and the consumption of palm oil is also increasing.

Palm oil is used chiefly for the manufacture of soaps and candles. It consists principally of palmitin and olein. Nordlinger * says that 98 per cent of the solid, fatty acids of palm oil is palmitic acid. The fresh oil has an agreeable odor, a bright orange color, and a consistency somewhat like that of butter. It is used as an edible fat by the natives of Africa.

Palm-kernel oil has a white or slightly yellow color. It has a composition which is quite different from palm oil and resembles coconut oil in its general composition, but contains a somewhat lower proportion of the glycerides of the lower fatty acids. The better grades are used for making vegetable butter, and the lower grades for soap manufacture.

The oil palm occurs naturally in immense numbers along the west coast of Africa. According to Hubert † the annual exports of oil and kernels from tropical Africa exceed in value forty million dollars. The oil palm grows well in the Philippine Islands and apparently produces fruit abundantly. It is not known to be attacked by any insects, fungi, or bacteria. Large plantations of oil palms are now being started in Sumatra and the Malay Peninsula. The cultivation of this plant in some parts of the Philippines would probably be advisable.

Family HERNANDIACEAE

Genus HERNANDIA

HERNANDIA OVIGERA (*peltata*) L.   Koron-kóron.

Local names: *Koron-kóron* (Camarines); *pantog-lóbo* (Tayabas).

HERNANDIA OVIGERA OIL

According to Heyne,‡ a fat used in lamps and for making candles is obtained from the fruits.

Hernandia ovigera is a small to medium-sized tree. The

---

* Nordlinger, Zeitschrift für angewandte Chemie, 1892, page 111.

† Hubert, P., Le palmier á huile.

‡ Heyne, K., De Nuttige Planten van Nederlandsch-Indië, Volume 2 (1916), page 177.

leaves are alternate, pointed at the tip, and frequently have the petiole attached within the margin. The flowers are whitish and about 1 centimeter wide.

This species is distributed from Luzon to Mindanao, but is apparently not common.

Family MORINGACEAE

Genus MORINGA

MORINGA OLEIFERA Lam.   MALUNGGÁI or HORSE-RADISH TREE.

Local names: *Arunggái* (Pangasinan); *balunggái* (Cuyo Islands); *kalamunggái* (Misamis); *kalunggái* (Camarines); *kamalunggái* (Mindoro); *kamalunggi* (Pampanga); *malugái* (Culion Island); *malunggái* (Tarlac, Bulacan, Zambales, Bataan, Rizal, Laguna, Manila, Batangas, Tayabas, Mindoro, Capiz, Zamboanga); *marunggái* (Ilocos Norte and Sur, Abra); *maronggói* (Zambales).

BEN OIL

The root of this species has a taste somewhat like that of horse-radish and in India is eaten by Europeans as a substitute for it. The wood, when fresh, has a like taste and odor. This species yields seeds from which ben oil is obtained.

The oil is said to be used for salads and culinary purposes, and to equal the best Florence oil as an illuminant. According to the bulletin of the Imperial Institute:*

The oil is particularly valuable for ointments since it can be kept for almost any length of time without undergoing oxidation. This property, together with the absence of colour, smell and taste, renders it peculiarly adapted for use in the "enfleurage" process of extracting perfumes.

The seeds of *Moringa oleifera* consist of about 8 per cent of husks and 92 per cent of kernels. The shelled kernels yield about 36 per cent of ben oil, which is obtained by expression. Table 10 shows the constants of cold- and hot-pressed oil obtained from Nigerian ben seeds.† Analyses of the oil cake which is left after expelling the oil from the ben seeds are given in Table 11.

TABLE 10.—*Constants of ben oil.*

Constants.	Crude cold-pressed oil from northern Nigeria.	Crude hot-pressed oil from northern Nigeria.
Specific gravity	0.9018	0.8984
Acid value	49.71	100.50
Saponification value	179.20	178.70
Unsaponifiable matter	1.67	2.69
Iodine value	100.30	88.00

* Bulletin of the Imperial Institute. Volume 2 (1904), page 118.
† Bulletin of the Imperial Institute. Volume 6, 1908, page 359.

TABLE 11.—*Analysis of oil cake from ben seeds.*

Constituents.	Hot-pressed cake, northern Nigeria.	Cake from Jamaica seed.
	Per cent.	*Per cent.*
Moisture	5.96	7.15
Albuminoids	24.12	21.51
Other nitrogenous substances	34.81	24.56
Fat	11.27	11.27
Fibre	4.32	
Ash	5.66	4.98
Other non-nitrogenous substances	13.86	

Ben oil consists largely of the glycerides of oleic, palmitic, and stearic acids. It also contains a solid acid of high melting point.

Moringa oleifera is a small tree 8 meters or less in height, with very soft, white wood and corky bark. The leaves are alternate, 25 to 50 centimeters long, and usually thrice pinnate. There are three to nine leaflets on the ultimate pinnules. The leaflets are 1 to 2 centimeters long. The pod is 15 to 30 centimeters long, pendulous, three-angled, and nine-ribbed. The seeds are three-angled and winged on the angles.

This species is widely distributed in the Philippines and in the tropics generally. It grows rapidly even in poor soil and is but little affected by drought.

Family PITTOSPORACEAE

Genus PITTOSPORUM

PITTOSPORUM PENTANDRUM (Blanco) Merr. MAMÁLIS.

Local names: *Balingkauáyan* (Antique); *basuít* (Abra); *bolongkoyan, saboágon* (Guimaras Island); *darayau* (Palawan); *dili* (Nueva Vizcaya); *lasuít, pasguik* (Benguet); *mamales* (Benguet, Rizal); *mamális* (Pangasinan, Bataan, Nueva Ecija, Bulacan, Rizal, Laguna); *oplái* (Iloko); *pañganto-an* (Cebu); *taliu* (Zambales).

MAMÁLIS OIL

Concerning the oil from this species, Bacon [*] writes:

* * * The fruits are quite small, and there is considerable labor involved in gathering them. One tree yielded 16 kilos of fruit which after grinding gave 210 cubic centimeters of an oil of pleasant odor by distillation with steam. The crude oil boiled from 153° to 165° and after being washed with alkalies and distilled over sodium, had the following properties:

---

[*] Bacon, R. F., Philippine terpenes and essential oils, III. Philippine Journal of Science, Section A, Volume 4 (1909), page 118.

Boiling point, 155° to 160° (principally 157° to 160°); specific gravity, $30°=0.8274$; $N\frac{30°}{D}=1.4620$; $A\frac{30°}{D}=40.40$.

These properties leave little doubt but that this oil consists principally of the same dihydroterpene that is found in the higher boiling portions of the oil of the ordinary petroleum nut.

Pittosporum pentandrum is a tree reaching a height of 20 meters and a diameter of about 50 centimeters. It is, however, usually much smaller than this. The leaves are alternate, pointed at both ends, about 10 centimeters long and less than 2 centimeters in width. The flowers are small, white, fragrant, and are crowded on small flowering branches. The fruits are about a centimeter long and contain a number of seeds.

This species is common and widely distributed in the Philippines from Luzon to Mindanao, especially in thickets and second-growth forests. Experiments have shown that it grows vigorously in cultivation.

PITTOSPORUM RESINIFERUM Hemsl. (Fig. 38).   PETROLEUM NUT.

Local names: *Abkol, abkel, lañgis* (Benguet); *dingo* (Mountain Province); *sagága* (Abra).

PETROLEUM-NUT OIL

The fruits of this species are known in the Philippines as petroleum nuts because of the fancied resemblance of the odor of the oil to that of petroleum and because even the green fresh fruits will burn brilliantly when a match is applied to them.

The chemical properties of the oil have been investigated by Bacon.* He found that the oil from the petroleum nut was very interesting, as it contained a dihydroterpene, $C_{10}H_{18}$, and also considerable quantities of normal heptane, which had only once before been found in nature, occurring in the digger pine (*Pinus sabiniana* Dougl.) of California.

In working up the various lots of *Pittosporum* fruits, considerable differences were noted in the proportion of heptane and dihydroterpene found in the oil, and the season and degree of ripeness of the fruits undoubtedly play a considerable rôle in this respect.

The first lot of nuts was obtained from Baguio, Benguet, in the autumn of 1907. One kilo of whole, fresh nuts gave 52 grams of oil on a press. The residue ground up and again pressed yielded an additional 16 grams of oil; specific gravity=0.883; $N\frac{30°}{D}=1.4577$. It was not possible to determine the optical rotation. The oil is quite sticky, and in a thin layer rapidly becomes resinous. In an open dish it burns strongly, with a sooty flame. It distills unchanged up to 165°, then with decomposition to give

* Bacon, R. F., Philippine terpenes and essential oils, III. Philippine Journal of Science, Section A, Volume 4 (1909), page 115.

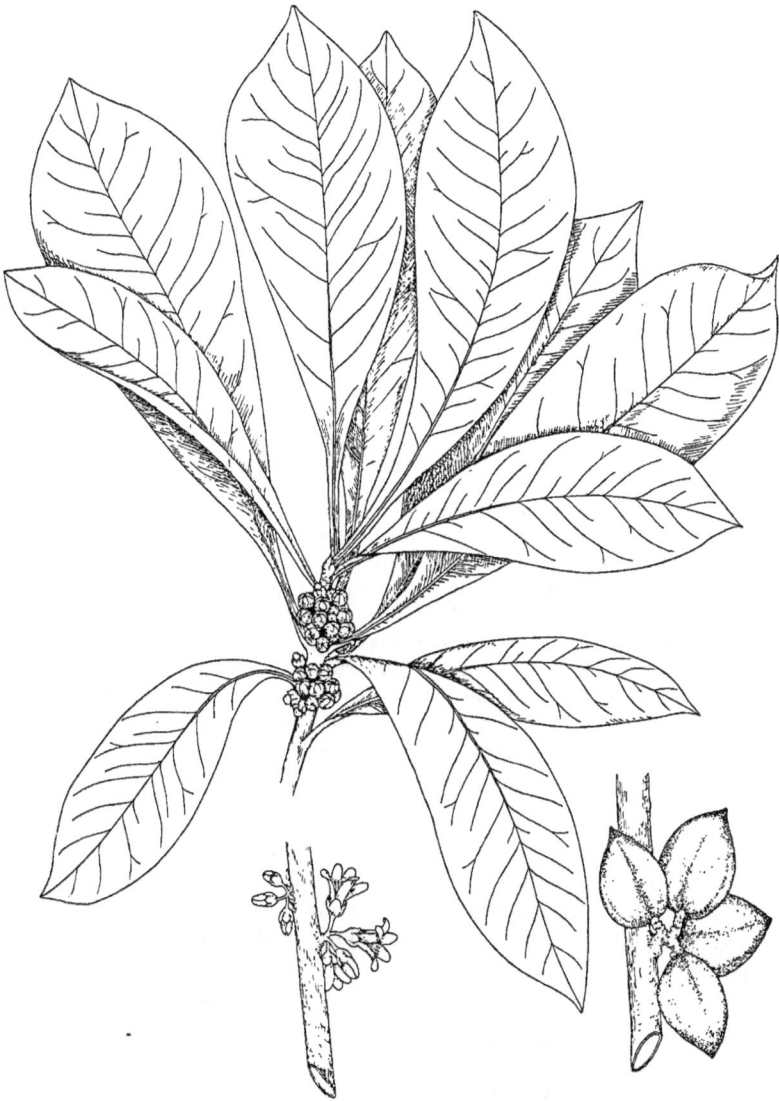

FIGURE 38. PITTOSPORUM RESINIFERUM (PETROLEUM NUT), THE SOURCE OF OIL OF
PETROLEUM NUTS. ×⅜.

a resin oil. The oil distilling from 100° to 165° is colorless, with an orange-like odor; specific gravity, $\frac{30°}{4}=0.7692$; $A\frac{30}{D}=+37°.0$. By two careful distillations the following fractions were obtained:

	Fraction (degrees.)	Grams.
(1)	98–103	41
(2)	103–110	18
(3)	110–120	21
(4)	120–140	12
(5)	140–150	7
(6)	150–155	47
(7)	155–160	49

Fraction No. 1 had a pleasant odor recalling oranges, and the following properties: specific gravity, $\frac{25°}{4}=0.6831$; $N\frac{D}{30°}=1.3898$; optical rotation=0.

Fraction No. 7 had a turpentine-like odor. Specific gravity, $\frac{30°}{4}=0.8263$, $N\frac{30°}{D}=1.4630$.

The properties of fraction No. 1 leave little doubt of the identity of this compound with normal heptane.

A second lot of petroleum nuts was obtained in December, 1908, from one of the upper ridges of Mount Mariveles, Bataan Province. One tree gave 15 kilos of fruits, which by pressure yielded 800 cubic centimeters of oil. The residue ground up and distilled with steam yielded 73 cubic centimeters more. This oil distilled in steam contained no heptane, showing that probably all the latter is in the oil cavities immediately surrounding the seeds, and that the pulp of the fruit contains only resins and the higher boiling portions of the oil. It was also noted that the leaves, branches, bark, wood, and in fact, all parts of the tree are distinctly resiniferous and have the same pleasant, orange-like odor as the fruits. * * *

Pittosporum resiniferum is a tree reaching a height of 25 to 30 meters, although in many cases it fruits when not over 6 to 12 meters high. It has fragrant, white flowers, about 1.3 centimeters long, which are borne in clusters on the stem. The leaves are smooth, pointed at both ends, and usually between 8 and 15 centimeters in length. The fruits are about 3 centimeters long.

This species is not very abundant in any part of the Islands, but is widely distributed and usually found on high mountain ridges.

Family LEGUMINOSAE

Genus ARACHIS

ARACHIS HYPOGAEA L.   Maní or Peanut.

PEANUT OIL

This plant is rather extensively grown in the Philippines and yields the edible nuts known as peanuts or ground nuts, from which arachis oil (peanut or ground-nut oil) is obtained by expression. High-grade arachis oil is nearly colorless and has a pleasant taste. It is edible and is used as a salad oil, especially as a cheaper substitute for olive oil. The lower grades are used for making soaps or for burning.

Very little peanut oil is produced in the Philippine Islands, but its manufacture on a large scale is well worth consideration, as in certain other countries it is an article of considerable commercial importance.

According to Thorpe,* the total quantity of arachis nuts produced in the world is approximately 350,000 tons per year. Large quantities of these nuts are used in France, Austria, Germany, and the United States. Although about 50,000 tons of peanuts are grown yearly in the United States, the demand is greater than the supply and consequently large quantities of nuts are imported.

Concerning the manufacture of peanut oil, Lewkowitsch † states that the nuts are shelled by special machinery. The kernels, which contain 43 to 45 per cent of oil, are ground and the oil expressed from the ground material by hydraulic pressure, two and sometimes three times. The first expression is carried out at the ordinary temperature, the second at about 31° C., and the third at about 52° C.

The cake serves as an excellent cattle food, as it contains the highest amount of proteins of all known oil cakes; moreover, these proteins are more easily digested than those of other cakes.

Thorpe † states that the average composition of the nuts obtained from various places is as follows:

	Per cent.
Arachis oil	38 to 50
Water	4.6 to 12.8
Albuminoids	26 to 31
Carbohydrates	5 to 19
Fibre	1.1 to 4.1
Ash	1.6 to 3.0

Mitchell ‡ gives the following constants for peanut oil:

Specific gravity	0.917 to 0.9256
Reichert-Meissl value	0.48
Hehner value	95.5
Iodine value	92 to 100.8

The principal fats which peanut oil contains are olein, linolin, palmitin, stearin, arachidin, and lignocerin.

* Thorpe, E., Dictionary of applied chemistry. Volume 1, page 286.
† Lewkowitsch, J., Oils, fats, and waxes. Volume 2, page 304.
‡ Mitchell, C. A., Edible oils and fats. Page 58.

Genus PACHYRRHIZUS

PACHYRRHIZUS EROSUS (L.) Urb.   SINGKAMÁS.

Local names: *Hingkamás* (Cavite); *kamáh* (Zambales); *kamás* (Ilocos Norte and Sur, Abra, Pangasinan); *lakamás* (Pangasinan); *sikamás* (Pampanga); *sinkamás* or *singkamas* (Ilocos Norte and Sur, Cagayan, Pangasinan, Tarlac, Bulacan, Bataan, Rizal, Manila, Laguna, Tayabas, Cavite, Batangas, Camarines, Albay, Mindoro, Capiz); *tikamás* (Cuyo Island).

SINGKAMÁS OIL

Heyne * says that Greshoff found in the seeds 38.4 per cent of a colorless, limpid oil.

Pachyrrhizus erosus is a rather coarse, somewhat hairy, herbaceous vine. The leaves are compound with three leaflets, which are up to 15 centimeters in length and 20 centimeters in width. The flowers are pale blue or blue and white, 2 to 2.5 centimeters long, and borne in racemes which are up to 45 centimeters in length. The pods are about 10 centimeters long, 10 to 12 millimeters wide, flat, hairy, and contain from eight to ten seeds. The roots are large, fleshy, turnip-shaped. They are either eaten raw or prepared in a variety of ways. The young fruit is sometimes eaten as a vegetable.

This species is a native of tropical America, but is now widely distributed in the tropics. It is thoroughly naturalized in the Philippines and is common in thickets. It is also extensively cultivated.

Genus PITHECOLOBIUM

PITHECOLOBIUM DULCE (Roxb.) Benth.   KAMACHÍLE.

KAMACHILE OIL

A description and the local names of this species are given in the bulletin on edible plants.

Concerning the oil yielded by the fruit of this species Kesava-Menon † states:

* * * The fruit * * * contains a number of large seeds each of which is enveloped in a sweet, whitish pulp. The seeds are black, shiny, partly immersed in an arillus, and replete with an edible pulp of an yellowish white colour. The pulp on extraction with ether yielded 18.22 per cent of a yellowish white oil, with a beany smell, which solidified at a temperature of 15° C. (=13.20 per cent calculated on the whole seed). The expressed oil is yellowish white, and very viscous, and "stearine" deposits on standing. The kernels form 72.4 per cent of the seed. Church (Dictionary of the Economic Products of India, Watt, Vol. VI, Part I, page 282) states that 100 parts of bean contain: water,

---

† Heyne, K., De Nuttige Planten van Nederlandsch-Indië, Volume 2 (1916), page 346.

† Kesava-Menon, A., Some Indian oils and fats. Journal of the Society of Chemical Industry, Volume 29 (1910), No. 24, page 1431.

13.5 parts; albuminoids, 17.67 parts; starch, 41.4 parts; fatty matter, 17.1 parts; fibre, 7.8 parts; ash, 2.6 parts.

Physical and chemical characteristics of Pithecolobium dulce—

Fat: Specific gravity (d 100/100) = 0.9106; (d 100/15) = 0.8756. Acid value, 63.9. Saponification value, 205.9. Reichert-Meissl value, 8.41. Titration no. of insol. vol. acids, 1/10 KOH, 0.34. Iodine value, 56.60. Unsaponifiable matter per cent, 1.17. Butyro-refractometer at 25° C. "Degrees," 69.5; at 40° C., 62.0.

Fatty acids: Per cent, 87.64. Melting point, 44.7° C. Iodine value, 57.59; neutralization value, 198.7. Mean molecular weight, 282.2.

Genus PONGAMIA

PONGAMIA PINNATA (*P. mitis*) (Linn.) Merr. (Fig. 39). BÁNI.

Local names: *Balobaló* (Zamboanga, Basilan); *balik-balík* (Tagalog); *baluk-balúk, balutbalút, magit* (Cotabato); *baobaó* (Agusan); *báni* (Pangasinan, Zambales, Pampanga, Bataan, Cotabato); *kadéi* (Tayabas); *marokbarók* (Bikol); *salingkugi* (Zamboanga).

PONGAM OIL

The seeds of this tree yield a red-brown, thick oil known as pongam oil. It is employed for illuminating and medicinal purposes and should also be useful for the manufacture of soap and candles. According to Lewkowitsch * the oil has the following constants:

Specific gravity at 40°... 0.9352
Saponification value 178.0
Iodine value 94.0
Refraction index at 40° (butyro refractometer degrees) 78.0

Concerning this oil Watt † says:

According to Lepine (*Pharm. Journ.* (*3*) *XL., 16*), the seeds yield 27 per cent of a yellow oil, having a sp. gr. of 0.945 and solidifying at 8°C. It has been examined by the authors of the *Pharmacographia Indica*, who write: "The oil which we have examined (called *Houge* oil in Mysore), and expressed purposely from fresh seeds, was thick, of a light orange-brown colour, and bitter taste. The sp. gr. at 18°C was 0.9458. It yielded 93.3 per cent of fatty acids melting at about 30°. With sulphuric acid it became yellow with orange streaks, and when stirred formed an orange-red mixture, which, after standing, became yellow. With nitric acid it formed an orange emulsion. With the elaïdin test it remained liquid for several hours, and was of the colour and consistence of honey after two days. The fresh oil deposits solid white fats if kept at the temperature of 16° for a few weeks, and the clear oil then has the specific gravity of 0.935. The bitter principle of the oil appears to reside in a resin, and not in an alkaloid as is the case with Margosa oil.

Pongamia pinnata is a tree reaching a height of 15 meters

---

* Lewkowitsch, J., Oils, fats, and waxes, Volume 2 (1915), page 498.

† Watt, G., A dictionary of the economic products of India, Volume 6 (1892), page 323.

and a diameter of about 45 centimeters. The leaves are alternate and compound with three to seven leaflets, which are
smooth, pointed at the apex, usually rounded at the base, and 7
to 10 centimeters in length. The flowers are purplish, about
1.5 centimeters in length, and borne in racemes. The pods are
somewhat flattened, somewhat oval in outline, and with a single
seed.

This species is distributed from northern Luzon to southern
Mindanao.

Genus TAMARINDUS

TAMARINDUS INDICA L.   SAMPÁLOK.

TAMARIND-SEED OIL

A description, figure, and the local names of this species are
given in the bulletin on edible plants.

Lewkowitsch * says that in famine times the seeds are univer-
sally eaten by the poorer classes of India, and that they yield
4.5 per cent of oil which has the following constants:

Saponification value... 183
Iodine value... 87.1

Hefter † states that the seeds yield 15 per cent of oil.
According to Watt: ‡

An oil of an amber colour, free of smell and sweet to the taste, is
prepared from the seeds by expression. This oil appears to have been
brought to notice for the first time in 1856, when a Captain Davies sent ‹
a sample to the Agri.-Horticultural Society of India, with the remark
that it was, in his opinion, suitable for culinary purposes. The Society's
Sub-Committee reported favourably on the oil, and suggested that it
might be found useful in the preparation of varnishes and paints, as well
as for burning in lamps. A member of the Committee remarked that it
was occasionally employed in Bengal for making a varnish to paint idols,
and for finishing *kurpa* cloth, but that it was very little appreciated. ‹
The Sub-Committee further noticed that the sample submitted to them
had an odour of linseed-oil, but Captain Davies explained that this was
not a property of the oil itself, but was due to the mill in which it had
been expressed, having been one ordinarily employed for making linseed-
oil (*Agri.-Hort. Soc. Ind., Journ., 1885*). The authors of the *Pharmacographia Indica* have examined it, and write, "Braunt states that the seeds
contain 20 per cent of a thickly fluid oil with an odour of linseed, and
classes it with the non-drying oils. By expression from the dry seeds,
we were unable to obtain any oil, and by solvents the yield was only 3.9
per cent. The oil possessed greater siccative properties than boiled linseed
oil." The subject appears to be well worthy of further investigation,

---

* Lewkowitsch, J., Chemical technology and analysis of oils, fats, and
waxes, Volume 2 (1914), page 238.

† Hefter, G., Technologie der Fette und Öle (1908), Volume 2, page 466.

‡ Watt, G., Dictionary of the economic products of India, Volume 6, Part
3 (1893), page 405.

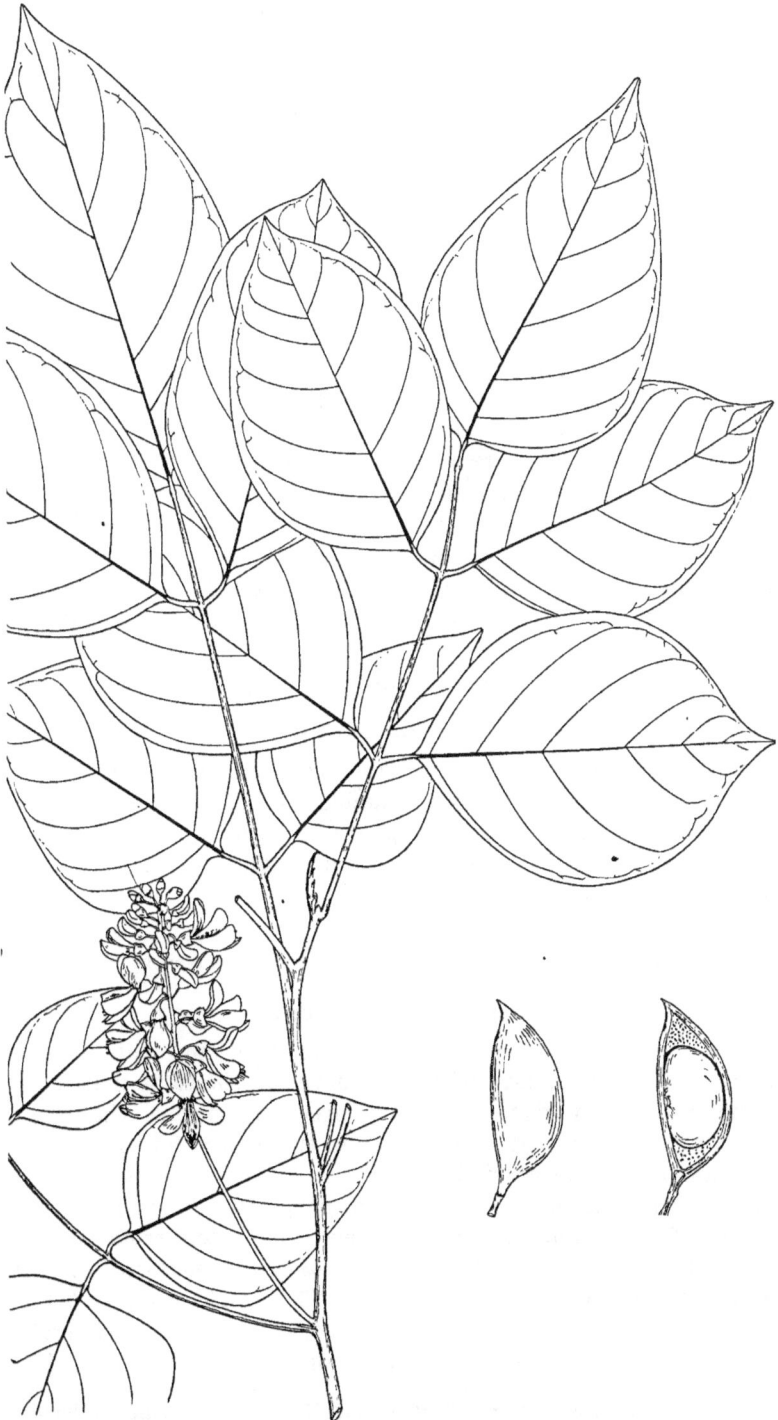

FIGURE 39. PONGAMIA PINNATA (BÁNI), THE SOURCE OF PONGAM OIL. ×⅓.

the more so from the contradictory nature of the literature regarding it, for the seeds might be obtained in any quantity and cheaply, should the oil prove of commercial value.

Family SIMARUBACEAE

Genus SAMADERA

SAMADERA INDICA Gaertn. MANUNGGÁL.

Local names: *Malunggál* (Mindoro); *manunggál* (Cagayan, Lanao).

MANUNGGÁL OIL

Heyne * says that Greshoff reports an oil content of one-third of the weight of the seed kernels. Heyne also states that the plant bears fruits in three years.

Samadera indica is a tree reaching a height of about 10 meters and a diameter of about 20 centimeters. The leaves are alternate, leathery, somewhat oval, pointed at both ends, and from 12 to 20 or more centimeters in length. The fruits are about 6 centimeters long, flattened, and inequilateral.

This species is distributed from Luzon to Mindanao and Palawan, but is apparently rare.

Family BURSERACEAE

Genus CANARIUM

Several species of the genus *Canarium* bear edible nuts which have a fine flavor and yield a valuable oil. The nuts are known as pili nuts. The largest are apparently produced by *Canarium ovatum* and these nuts are sold commercially as pili.

CANARIUM OVATUM Engl. (Fig. 40). PÍLI.

Local names: *Anánggi* (Sorsogon); *basiád, lipúti, piláuai* (Tayabas); *piláui* (Polillo); *píli* (Tayabas, Polillo, Camarines, Sorsogon, Samar, Surigao).

PILI NUTS AND PILI-NUT OIL

The nuts of this species are very rich in oil, and when roasted have a delicious flavor. They are served in the same manner as almonds, and by many are considered superior to the latter. The nuts are also used considerably in the making of confections. In Camarines, the roasted kernels are used to adulterate chocolate. The uncooked nuts have a purgative effect. In 1913, 1,186,173 kilograms of pili nuts were exported from Manila. The oil obtained from the nuts of *Canarium ovatum* is sweet, and suitable for culinary purposes. The fruits are 6 to 7 centimeters in length and consist of hard, thick-shelled, triangular nuts surrounded by a small amount of pulp. This pulp, which

---

* Heyne, K., De Nuttige Planten van Nederlandsch-Indië, Volume 3 (1917), page 23.

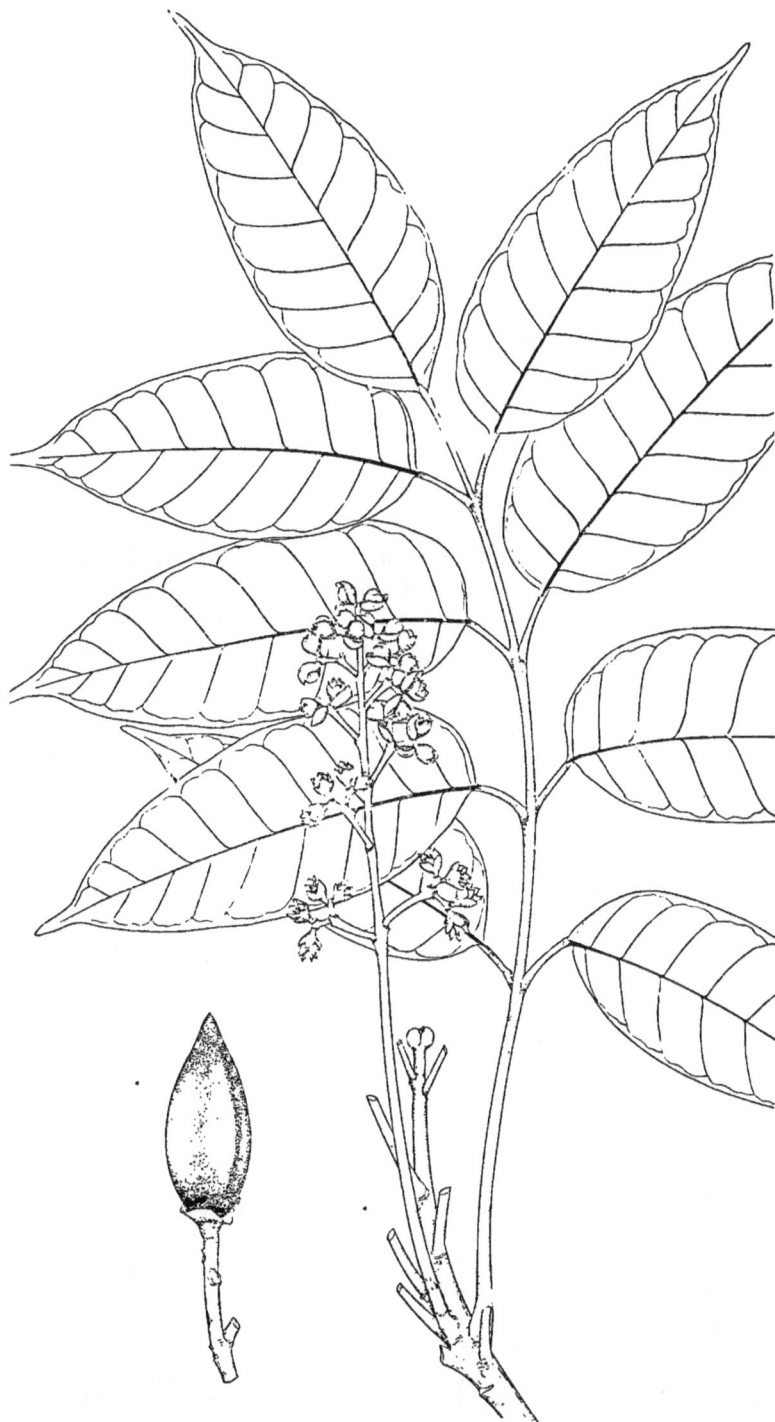

FIGURE 40. CANARIUM OVATUM (PĪLI), THE SOURCE OF PĪLI-NUT OIL.
168837—8

is edible when cooked, also contains an oil which is occasionally extracted locally and used for lighting and in cooking. Its chemical properties have not been investigated.

Mr. E. Tabat, who kept a record of the yield of a number of trees, found that an average tree produced 33 kilos of nuts in one year. The cost of gathering the nuts was 2.5 centavos per kilo, and of husking them, 1.5 centavos per kilo.

Mr. Tabat tried three methods of removing the soft covering of the nuts and found that the best method was to place them in fresh water for at least 24 hours, after which the soft part was easily removed. If the fresh nuts were put in sacks and piled in a corner and the soft covering allowed to rot, many of the nuts were spoiled, apparently by the heat produced by the decay of the soft, outer coverings. This method also resulted in the loss of sacks. He found it inadvisable to remove the soft covering by means of hot water, as this frequently cooked the nuts, thus greatly impairing their keeping qualities.

Brill and Agcaoili * analyzed what they called long and short varieties of pili nuts from *Canarium pachyphyllum*. The results are recorded in Tables 12 and 13.

TABLE 12.—*Composition of the kernels of pili nuts.*

	Long.	Short.
	Per cent.	Per cent.
Moisture	2.79	2.90
Fat	74.39	72.53
Protein (N x 6.25)	12.06	11.88
Sucrose	0.88	0.66
Reducing sugars	0.45	1.35
Starch (by difference)	4.33	5.11
Crude fiber	2.15	2.42
Ash	2.97	3.15

TABLE 13.—*Chemical constants of pili oil.*

	Long.	Short.
Specific gravity at 30° C	0.9067	0.9067
Butyro refractometer reading at 30° C	54-54.2	54-54.2
Iodine value (Hanus)	61.25	59.61
Reichert-Meissl value	3.3	2.2
Saponification number	192.6	186.8
Free fatty acids (oleic) _____ per cent.	7.62	8.84
Acid value _____ cc. N/10 NaOH	2.70	3.13

* Brill, H. C., and Agcaoili, F., Philippine oil-bearing seeds and their properties: II. Philippine Journal of Science, Section A, Volume 10 (1915), page 110.

This species, like *Canarium luzonicum*, yields Manila elemi, for a discussion of which see *Canarium luzonicum*, in the section on resins.

Canarium ovatum is a tree reaching a height of about 20 meters and a diameter of about 40 centimeters. The leaves are alternate and compound with opposite leaflets, which are smooth, rounded at the base, pointed at the tip, and from 10 to 20 centimeters in length. The flowers are greenish, fragrant, and about a centimeter long.

This species is very abundant in southern Luzon.

Family MELIACEAE

Genus CHISOCHETON

CHISOCHETON CUMINGIANUS Harms. (Fig. 41).   BALUKANÁG.

Local names: *Balita* (Bukidnon sub-province;) *balukanág* (Laguna, Camarines, Catanduanes Island); *batuákan* (Benguet, Union); *bayongbói* (Nueva Vizcaya); *diualat* (Tayabas); *dudós* (Albay); *kalimotáin* (Laguna); *káto* (Bataan); *makalsa* (Negrito in Cagayan); *malakalád* (Negros Oriental); *maramabólo* (Cagayan); *pakalsa* (Cagayan); *salagin* (Laguna).

BALUKANÁG OIL

This species produces a nut averaging 3 centimeters in length and 2.5 centimeters in width. The nut contains a considerable percentage of non-drying oil. It is reported to have been, before petroleum became common, the chief source of illuminating oil in certain regions. The nuts have rather hard shells which, according to Brill and Agcaoili,* constitute about 60 per cent of the total weight of the seed and are somewhat difficult to separate from the meat. They found that 1 kilogram of shelled nuts after drying weighed 698 grams, and yielded by extraction with petroleum ether 308 grams, or approximately 31 per cent of the fresh kernels, of a reddish-brown oil which had the specific gravity 0.9203 at 15.5° C.

The dried kernels had the following composition:

	Per cent.
Fat (by extraction)	44.12
Protein (N x 6.25)	9.00
Ash	3.19

By expression of the dried kernel, Brill and Agcaoili obtained 35.56 per cent of balukanág oil. According to them, the oil has a rancid odor, is non-drying, and has purgative properties. The laxative effect of 5 parts of this would be approximately equiva-

---

* Brill, H. C. and Agcaoili, F., Philippine oil-bearing seeds and their properties: II. Philippine Journal of Science, Section A, Volume 10 (1915), page 107.

lent to one part of castor oil. These writers state that the soap-making quality of this oil was tested by the Bureau of Science with gratifying results and that the oil is now being used by at least one firm in Manila in this industry.

Balukanág oil has the following chemical constants:

Specific gravity at 15° C..	0.9203
Specific gravity at 30° C..	0.9188
Butyro refractometer (reading at 30° C.)......................	60–61
Iodine value (Hanus)..	80.78
Reichert-Meissl value..	7.34
Saponification number..	192.02
Free fatty acids (oleic)...................................per cent....	3.98
Acid value..cc. N/10 KOH....	7.06

Chisocheton cumingianus is a tree reaching a height of 20 meters and a diameter of 45 centimeters. The flowers are fairly numerous, on long inflorescences. The leaves are compound with leaflets about 20 to 25 centimeters in length. The fruit is pear-shaped and when dry is about 8 centimeters in diameter. It contains nuts averaging 3 centimeters in length and 2.5 centimeters in width.

This species is distributed from northern Luzon to Mindanao.

CHISOCHETON PENTANDRUS (Blco.) Merr. (Fig. 42).   KÁTONG-
MACHÍN.

Local names: *Igíu* (Tayabas); *kátong-bakálau, malatumbága, kátong-machín* (Bataan); *pamalat'áñgen* (Cagayan).

KÁTONG-MACHÍN OIL

Oil extracted from the fruit of this species is used locally as a hair cosmetic.

Chisocheton pentandrus is a tree reaching a height of 30 meters and a diameter of 40 centimeters. The leaves are alternate and compound. The leaflets are opposite, pointed at the tip, rounded at the base, and 7 to 14 centimeters in length. The flowers are small and are borne on long-branched inflorescences. The fruits are round, red, hairy, and about 1.5 centimeters in diameter.

This species is distributed throughout the Archipelago.

Genus **XYLOCARPUS**

XYLOCARPUS MOLUCCENSIS Lam.   PIAGÁU.

PIAGÁU OIL

A description and figure of this species and its local names are given in the bulletin on mangrove swamps.

Heyne * says that, according to Wijs, the seeds contain 40 to

* Heyne, K., De Nuttige Planten van Nederlandsch-Indië, Volume 3 (1917), page 45.

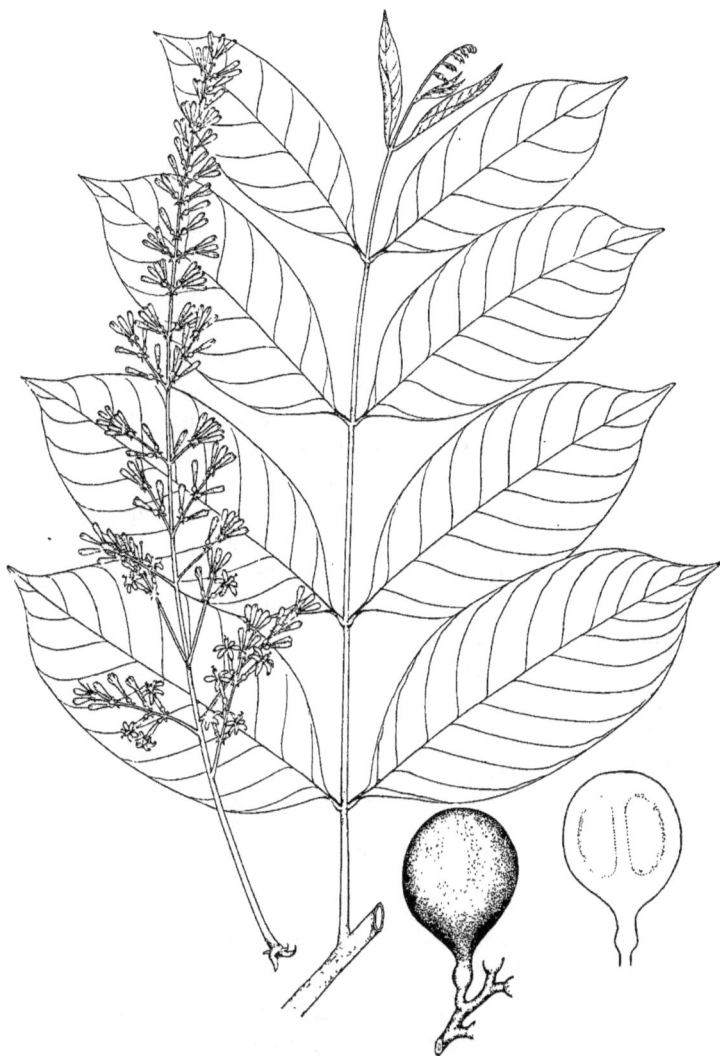

FIGURE 41. CHISOCHETON CUMINGIANUS (BALUKANÁG), THE SOURCE OF BALUKA-
NÁG OIL. ×½.

60 per cent of solid fat with a strong, bitter taste, which can be removed by prolonged boiling with water. The odor is slightly acid and somewhat aromatic.

According to Watt: *

The seeds yield, on expression, a whitish semi-solid fat. This remains fluid only at high temperatures. It is used as a hair-oil, and also for burning purposes.

Family EUPHORBIACEAE

Genus ALEURITES

TUNG OIL AND LUMBANG OILS

This genus contains a number of species with nuts which yield a valuable oil. Perhaps the best known of these oils is Chinese wood oil or tung oil. This is derived from at least two Chinese species of the genus, *Aleurites fordii* Hemsley and *A. montana* Wilson, which do not occur in the Philippines. Tung oil, which has properties quite similar to those of the Philippine lumbang oils, has been investigated quite extensively, and for this reason a short account of this important oil has been included.

Tung oil is used in large quantities for the preparation of paints, varnishes, linoleum, and for other similar purposes. According to Brill and Agcaoili † 5,000,000 gallons of Chinese wood oil were imported from China into the United States in 1911. These writers state that 40,000 trees have been planted in the southern states by American paint concerns.

As regards the importance of tung oil, the Oil, Paint, and Drug Reporter ‡ states:

* * * In recent years this oil has revolutionized the varnish industry of the United States, for it has made possible the manufacture of a quick-drying varnish that is less liable to crack than that made from kauri gum. Tung oil has also been found of special value in waterproof priming for cement. * * *

EXTRACTION METHODS

The Chinese methods employed for extracting the oil, although crude, are effective. After the seeds are removed from the husks they are placed in a circular stone trough, where they are crushed by a stone roller drawn by a buffalo, cow, or ass. The pulverized meal is partially roasted in shallow pans, then steamed over boiling water, the product meantime

---

* Watt, G., Dictionary of the economic products of India, Volume 2 (1889), page 141.

† Brill, H. C. and Agcaoili, F., Philippine oil-bearing seeds and their properties: II. Philippine Journal of Science, Section A, Volume 10 (1915), page 113.

‡ Oil, Paint, and Drug Reporter, Volume 91, February 12, 1917, page 48L.

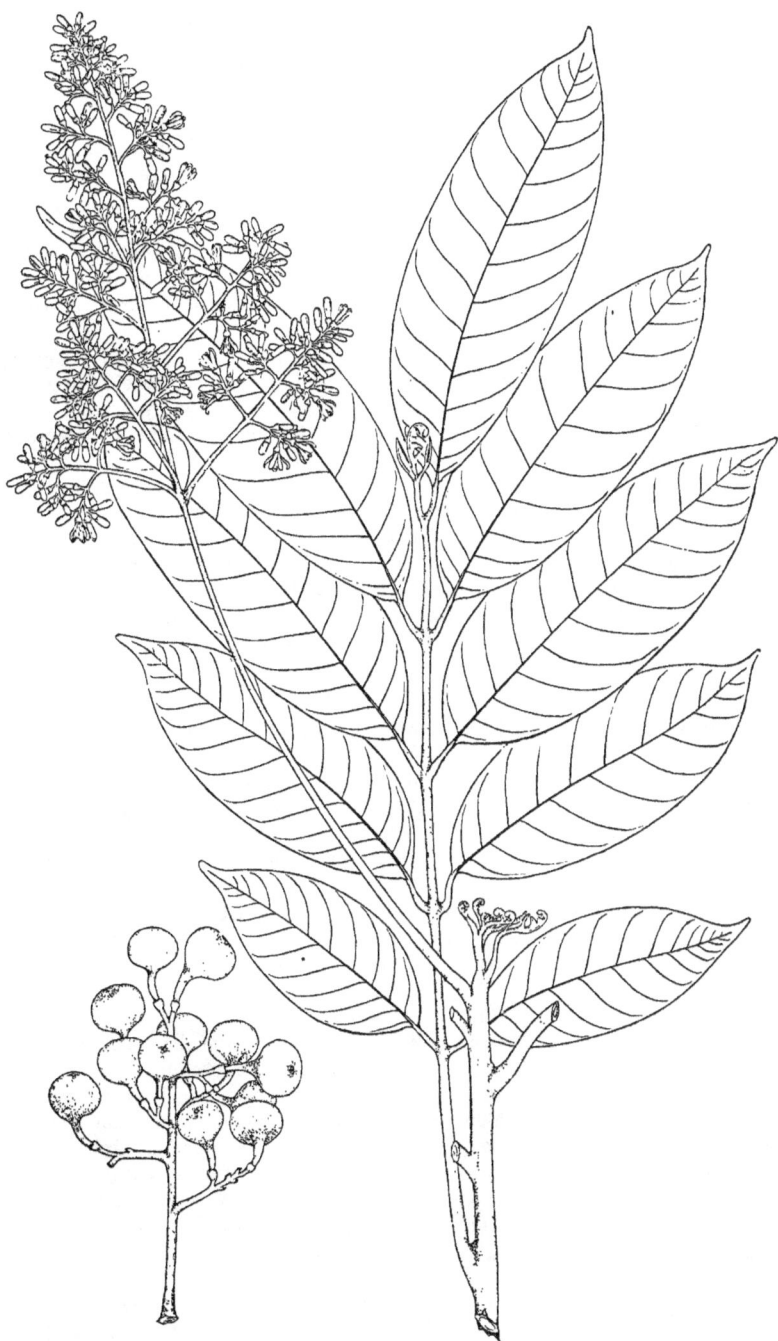

FIGURE 42. CHISOCHETON PENTANDRUS (KÁTONG-MACHIN), THE SOURCE OF KÁTONG-MACHÍN OIL. ×½

being placed in wooden vats fitted with wicker bottoms. The nuts are next placed in steel frames with straw as an outside container. The frames are arranged on edge in a press and pressure is applied. This is usually accomplished by means of a system of wedges which are driven in one after another by means of a huge battering-ram until the brown, watery, and odoriferous oil is crushed out into the vat below. As a rule the oil is then slightly heated and strained through a coarse grass cloth. (If the heating process is carried too far the oil becomes dark brown instead of retaining its desired light-yellow color.) The product is then placed in wicker baskets lined with varnished paper and is ready for shipment. As a rule the oil yield is about 40 per cent of the original weight of the kernels. The refuse matter, which is in the form of cakes, is used as a fertilizer.

In the vicinity of Hankow the native dealers allow the oil to again precipitate, drawing off the clear liquid and selling it to the foreign exporting firms. The residue is then sold to small dealers in Wuchang and Hanyang, who once more skim the oil after a further precipitation process. The oil is then sold to the native boatmen for use on their craft.

About the only variation in the above method of oil extraction is that in cold weather, when the oil congeals to a grease stage, it is necessary to heat the mass slightly in order to allow precipitation to take place. This is usually accomplished by steam coils being placed within the containing tank. Under this treatment the product soon liquifies, the foreign matter drops to the bottom, and the clear liquid is drained off through stopcocks placed just high enough to avoid the thick, muddy sediment at the bottom.

VARIED USES OF THE OIL

T'ung-yu is widely used throughout China as a paint oil for outside purposes. It is held that as a drying oil it excels even linseed oil. One of its greatest local markets is found among the native boatmen, who never paint their boats but coat them with the cruder grades of wood oil, which not only give the woodwork a bright, lustrous finish but also act as an excellent preservative. When certain mineral substances known as t'utzu and t'o-shen are added to the wood oil and the resulting mass heated for about two hours a varnish called kuang-yu is produced which is valuable as a water-proofing substance when placed on silks, pongees, and the like.

T'ung-yu is also used as an adulterant in the manufacture of lacquer varnish, as an illuminant, and as an ingredient in concrete, and when mixed with lime and bamboo shavings it is used by the natives in calking their boats. The so-called Chinese or Indian ink is made from the soot resulting from the burning of the oil or the fruit husks. The product is also used as a dressing for leather, in the manufacture of soap, and as a varnish for fine furniture. It is chiefly used in foreign countries for the manufacture of varnish from cheap gums. Other oils require a higher and more expensive quality of gum in order that the resulting varnish be of equal grade. This feature, together with the rapidity with which wood-oil varnish dries, has caused the demand for the product to steadily increase.

According to Ennis: *

China wood oil is rapidly becoming conspicuous as a linseed oil substitute in the varnish trade. * * * The consumption of the oil in the

---

* Ennis, W. D. Linseed oil and other oils (1909), page 235.

United States has been steadily increasing. There are two grades of the oil, one yellow and the other darker. * * * The oil is extremely poisonous and, as received from the Chinese, subject to heavy adulteration. * * * The crude oil dries with extreme rapidity, but with an opaque film, due to the presence of mucilaginous matter, which also causes the oil to become waxy at low temperatures, when organic compounds analogous to stearates settle out. It cannot be used in its raw state, but is always chemically treated. It may be "boiled" with lead or manganese dryers, with rosin or with resinates, to hasten oxidation, but must not be heated above 350 degrees F., at which temperature it suddenly thickens to an insoluble gelatine-like substance which cannot be softened again. It is nearly always used in a mixture with linseed oil. Its characteristic lard-like odor may be detected in solutions as weak as 10 per cent.

Brown * gives analyses and specifications of high-grade Chinese wood oil and also the correction factor for calculating the specific gravity at different temperatures.

Stevens of Irvington, N. J., and Armitage † of Newark, N. J., have compiled a very extensive bibliography of Chinese wood oil which they claim comprises the entire literature' on the subject. This is issued in two volumes, each consisting of two parts which are really volumes in themselves.

In the Philippines, oil is obtained from two species of this genus, *Aleurites moluccana* (lumbang) and *Aleurites trisperma* (bagilumbang). These oils have been studied by Brill and Agcaoili, who believe that either could be substituted for tung oil, as they are quick-drying and give a clear, transparent, nonsticking film on a surface when exposed to the air for a short time. If the Philippine oils are placed on the market, they will probably be used primarily for the same purposes as tung oil. The oil obtained from *Aleurites trisperma* is almost indistinguishable from tung oil for the uses which the latter chiefly serves, while that obtained from *Aleurites moluccana* is possibly slightly inferior to tung oil, although superior to linseed oil.

Tung oil heated to a temperature of about 200° to 250⁼ solidifies, and in this condition is unsuitable for making varnishes. We have found that oil from *Aleurites moluccana* or *A. trisperma* may be heated to about 315° at which temperature it distills and does not solidify until about one-third has been volatilized. In so far as this property is concerned the Philippine lumbang oils are more suitable for varnish making than is tung oil.

---

* Brown, F., Chemical News, Volume 114 (1916), page 123.

† Stevens, G. H., and Armitage, J. W., Patents, technology and bibliography of China wood oil (tung oil), 1914.

Aguilar,* who also has made a study of the Philippine oils, says that lumbang oil is similar to linseed oil in its properties as a paint vehicle, and that, like linseed, it has certain disadvantages for use in red-lead paints. Bagilumbang oil cannot be used as a paint vehicle, especially with red lead, as it dries into a paste. Aguilar found that a mixture of the two oils, containing 25 to 50 per cent of lumbang oil makes a good paint vehicle for red lead. The *Aleurites* oil so far produced in the Philippines is almost entirely the product of *Aleurites moluccana*, which is fairly abundant in a wild state in many parts of the Philippines, and is also planted. *Aleurites trisperma* is reported from many localities, but is probably not so abundant. Both species can be grown readily in plantations.

The Bureau of Forestry is using large numbers of both species in its reforestation projects and is also distributing seed and encouraging other people to plant these species. It is safe to say that at the present time the yearly planting of these species amounts to between 400,000 and 500,000 trees. From these figures it would seem reasonable to predict that in the near future large quantities of *Aleurites* oil will be available in the Philippines. During the year 1918, 184,428 kilograms of *Aleurites moluccana* oil valued at 129,838 pesos were exported from the Philippines.

That there would be a market for considerable quantities of *Aleurites moluccana* (lumbang) oil is shown by the fact that one American concern, which has experimented with this oil, has inquired as to the possibility of obtaining 4,000 tons per month.

ALEURITES MOLUCCANA (L.) Willd. (Figs. 43–45).   LUMBÁNG.

Local names: *Biáo* (Misamis, Davao); *lumbáng* (Rizal, Laguna, Zamboanga, Batangas); *lumbang-bató* (Cavite).

LUMBÁNG OIL.

The oil of *Aleurites moluccana* is known in the Philippines as lumbang oil. This species is distributed through Polynesia, the Malayan region, and the Hawaiian Islands. In Hawaii the oil is called kukui or candle-nut oil. The latter name is also used in other parts of the world. According to Wilcox and Thompson † the Hawaiians strung the nuts on sticks and used

---

* Aguilar, R. H., The lumbang oil industry in the Philippine Islands. Philippine Journal of Science, Volume 14 (1919), pages 275–285.

† Wilcox, E. V. and Thompson, A. R., The extraction and use of kukui oil. Hawaii Agricultural Experiment Station, Press Bulletin 39 (1913).

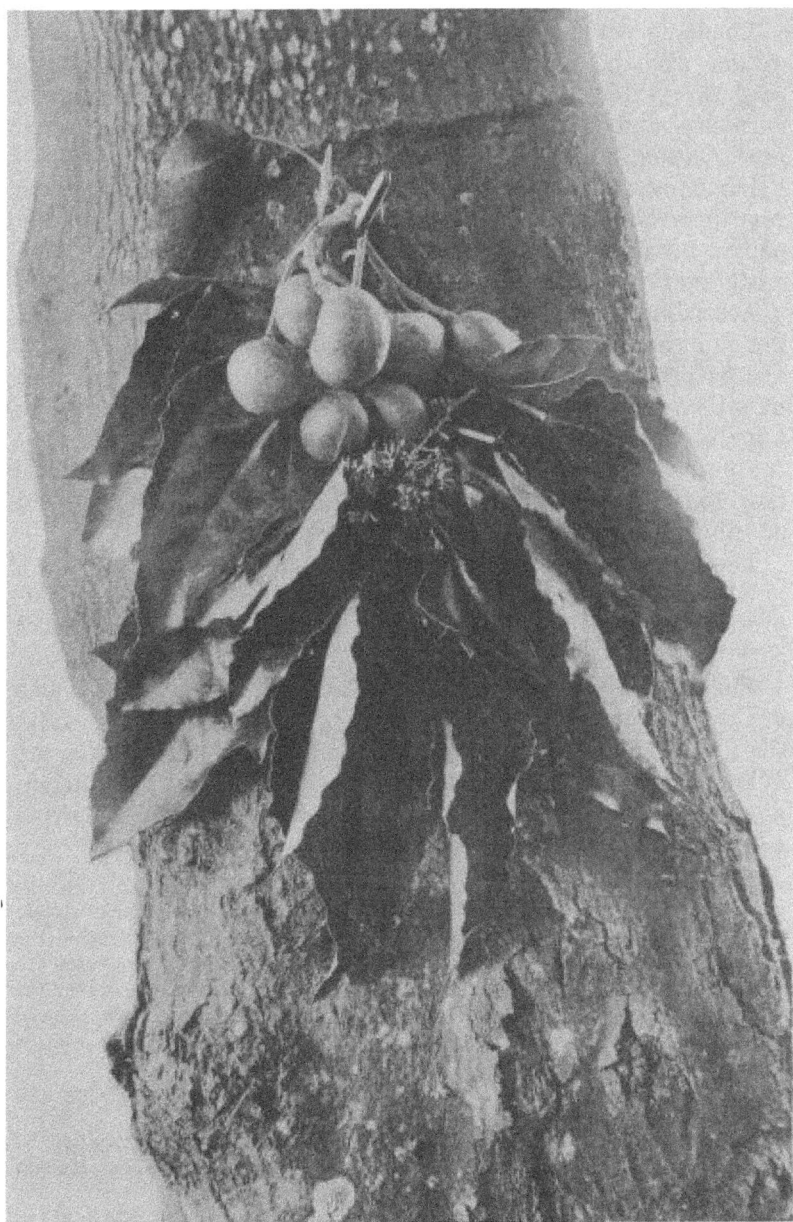

FIGURE 43. ALEURITES MOLUCCANA (LUMBÁNG), THE SOURCE OF LUMBÁNG OIL.
BARK, FRUITS, AND LEAVES.

them for lighting their houses. This use of the kernels gave rise to the name "candle nut."

Lumbang is a drying oil and in this respect resembles linseed oil and also the Chinese wood oil (tung oil). Lumbang oil is used for various purposes, such as the preparation of paints, varnishes and linoleum, illumination, soap manufacture, wood preservation, etc.

Lumbang oil has been manufactured in the Philippines in very primitive mills for years, and is used locally for mixing paints, for protecting bottoms of dugout canoes and other small craft against water and marine borers, and for illumination.

According to Richmond and Rosario,* who examined the Philippine nuts, the whole nuts are composed of 66 per cent of shells and 34 per cent of kernels, and the kernels contain 52 per cent of oil. Wilcox and Thompson † state that the whole nut contains 67 per cent of shells and 33 per cent of kernels, and that the kernels contain 60 per cent of oil. Lewkowitsch ‡ reports that some samples of lumbang kernels contain 62.25 per cent of oil and others 58.6 per cent.

The oil manufactured locally is made in a few Chinese shops in Manila, with primitive hand apparatus. The nuts are hot-pressed to save labor, but it is said that cold-pressing produces a better grade of oil.

The nuts of *Aleurites moluccana* have very hard shells which are difficult to crack; and, moreover, it is .difficult to separate the kernel from the shell. A common procedure is to crack the nuts and pick out the kernels by means of a pointed instrument, a very tedious operation. Aguilar § mentions the following methods which are also used to separate shell from kernel:

In some localities the Chinese place large quantities of nuts on the ground, cover them with straw and after burning the straw immediately sprinkle the nuts with cold water. They claim that with this method the nuts burst. In Laguna, Tayabas, and Batangas Provinces, the nuts are placed in tanks of boiling water and left there for from five to six hours. This loosens the kernel, and when sufficiently cool the nuts are cracked and the kernels are separated from the shells. These two methods produce brown kernels from which only brown oil can be expressed.

In Moro Province, along the coast of Davao, the nuts are dried in the

* Richmnd, G. F., and Rosario, M. V. del, Commercial utilization of some Philippine oil-bearing seeds: preliminary paper. Philippine Journal of Science, Volume 2 (1907), pages 439 to 449.

† Wilcox, E. V., and Thompson, A. R., The extraction and use of kukui oil. Hawaii Agricultural Experiment Station, Press Bulletin 39, (1913).

‡ Lewkowitsch, J. Oils, fats, and waxes (1915).

§ Aguilar, R. H., The lumbang oil industry in the Philippine Islands. Philippine Journal of Science, Volume 14 (1919), page 275.

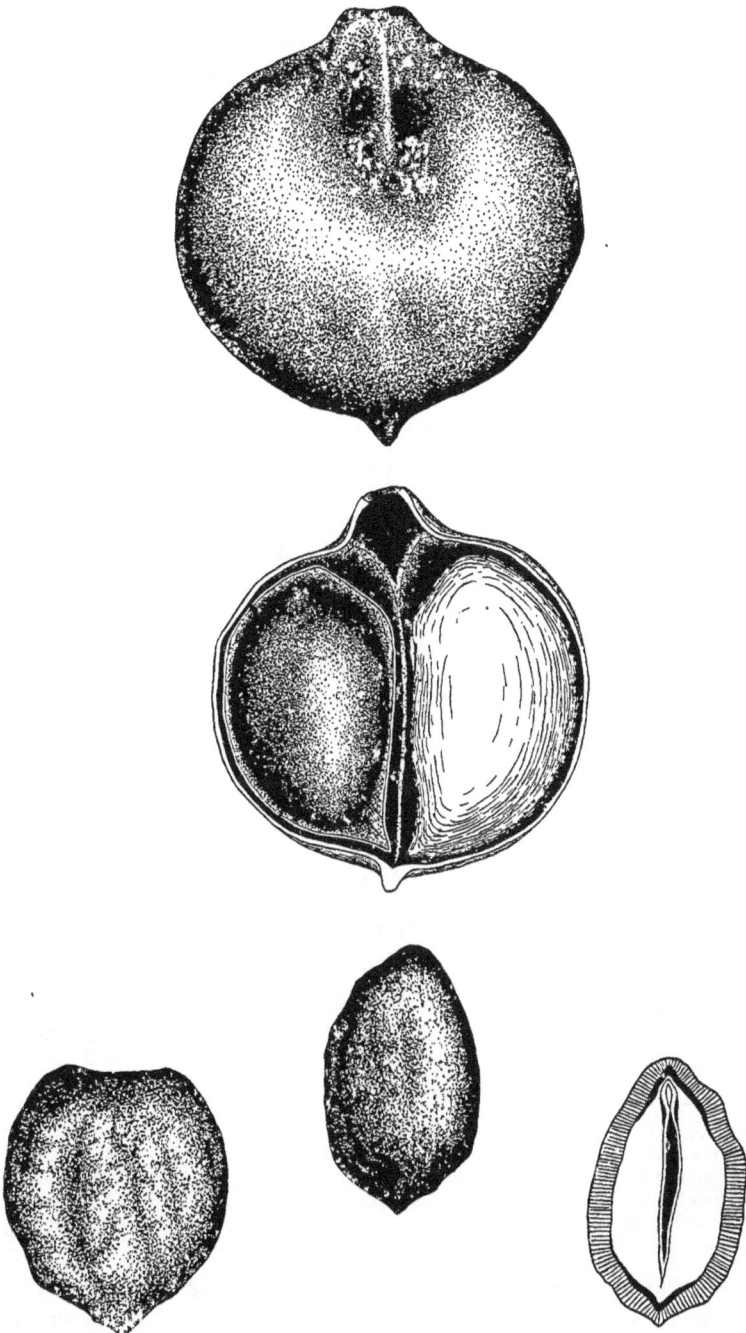

FIGURE 44. ALEURITES MOLUCCANA (LUMBÁNG), THE SOURCE OF LUMBÁNG OIL. DRIED FRUITS AND SEEDS. NATURAL SIZE.

sun until the kernels loosen sufficiently, which may be ascertained by occasionally cracking a few nuts for trial. The drying takes from five to ten days or more, depending upon the condition of the weather; the nuts are then cracked and the kernels removed. This process is very slow, although the kernel usually comes out whole and is of the best quality.

Aguilar has developed the following method: Nuts are heated in an oven at 95 degrees for three or four hours and then placed in cold water and left overnight. By the next morning most of the shells have burst and the kernels are picked out without much difficulty. This method, he says, has no injurious effect on the oil.

The following methods of removing the shells from the seeds are in practice in the Province of Laguna. The seeds are placed over a fire for from 72 to 120 hours, at the end of which time the shells are cracked, or they are spread in the sunshine until cracks are visible in the shells. In both cases, after the shells crack, the seeds are thrown against a hard object, preferably a large stone, when the shells fall off in pieces. These methods give brown kernels.

It has been suggested that the nuts with the shells could be crushed and ground in an oil mill and the oil expressed from the ground material. Aguilar believes, however, that the best method is to separate the kernel from the shell and then extract the oil; as about 20 kilos more oil per ton of nuts may be extracted from the kernel than from the crushed nuts. At present the Chinese manufacturers sell the cake, which is left after the oil is extracted from the nuts, at a good profit. According to the results obtained by Aguilar (Table 14), the fertilizing value of the cake left from the crushed nuts would be so much reduced as to make it almost useless as a fertilizer.

TABLE 14.—*Fertilizing value of lumbang (Aleurites moluccana) cake.*

Constituents.	Cake from kernel.	Cake from crushed nuts.
	Per cent.	*Per cent.*
Moisture	11.13	8.46
Nitrogen (N₂)	8.86	1.25
Potash (K₂O)	1.67	0.68
Phosphorous (P₂O₅)	1.02	0.25

Aguilar has found that the nuts of *Aleurites moluccana* may be stored a year or more without any appreciable change in the amount or composition of the oil. However, when the kernels without the shells are stored, they are apt to be very severely

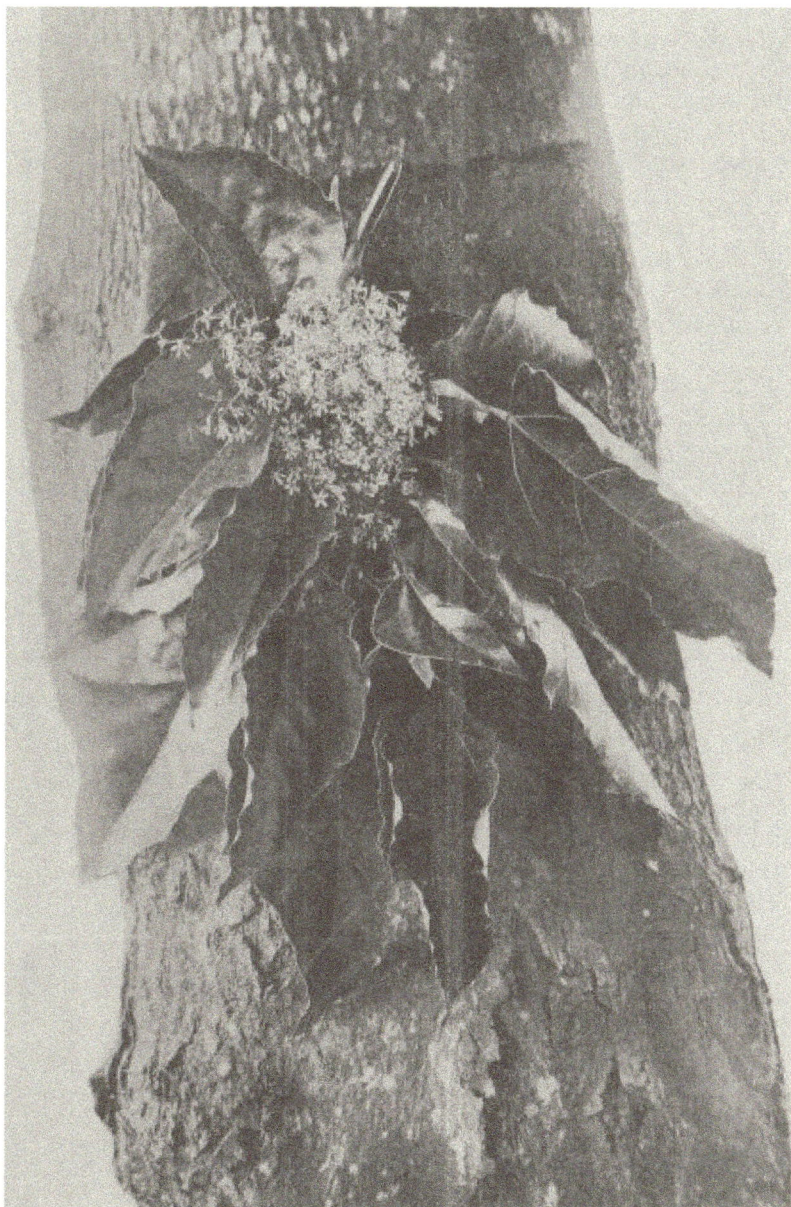

FIGURE 45. ALEURITES MOLUCCANA (LUMBÁNG), THE SOURCE OF LUMBÁNG OIL. BARK, FLOWERS, AND LEAVES.

attacked by small beetles, and the oil becomes more and more acid, although no change may be noticed in the appearance of the kernel and oil extracted. An actual test showed that the acidity of the oil was increased from 0.55 to 5.32 when the kernels were stored in a cold, dry place for one month. It is therefore advisable to extract the oil from fresh nuts.

Analyses of the kernels of *Aleurites moluccana* show that the principal constituents are oil (consisting largely of fat) and protein. The percentage of fiber and ash is very low. This is shown by the results recorded in Table 15.

TABLE 15.—*Analyses of lumbang kernels.*

Constituents.	Sample.	
	1.[a]	2.[b]
Water	5.00	8.23
Oil	62.175	59.93
Protein	22.65	8.04
Nitrogen free extract	6.83	17.62
Ash	3.345	3.56
Fiber		2.62

[a] Semler, H., Die Tropische Agrikultur, Volume 2, page 515.
[b] Agricultural Gazette, New South Wales, Volume 17, (1906), page 859.

Lumbang oil has a light yellow color, and an agreeable odor and taste. It dries in thin films when allowed to stand several days. The results of various analyses of lumbang oil quoted by Wilcox and Thompson are given in Table 16. Aguilar also analyzed various samples of lumbang oil. His results are given in Table 17.

TABLE 16.—*Constants of lumbang oil (Wilcox and Thompson).*

Constants.	Sample.				
	1.[a]	2.[b]	3.[c]	4.[d]	5.[e]
Specific gravity 15° C	0.925	0.920–0.926	0.925	0.925	0.924
Acid value	1.72			0.97	0.5
Saponification value	204.2	184–187.4	192.6	194.8	189.5
Iodine value	139.7	136.3–139.3	163.7	114.2	152.8
Hehner value	96.4		95.5		95.2
Volatile acids	1.98			1.2	
Titer	17.8				
Butyro-refractometer		76–75.5 (15°C)	76 (25°C)		

[a] Imperial Institute, Bulletin of Imperial Institute, Volume V (1907), page 135.
[b] De Negri, Journal of the Society of Chemical Industry, Volume XX (1901), page 909.
[c] Lewkowitsch, Journal of the Society of Chemical Industry, Volume XX (1901), page 909.
[d] Fendler, G., Journal of the Society of Chemical Industry, Volume XXIII (1904), page 613.
[e] Kassler, Journal of the Society of Chemical Industry, Volume XXII (1903), page 639.

TABLE 17.—*Constants of lumbang oil (Aguilar)*.

Constants.	Oil extracted from fresh kernels.	Oils obtained from the market.	
		Grade I.	Grade II.
Appearance	light colored	brown	dark brown
Sp. gr. at 15.5° C	0.9261	0.9253	0.9237
Saponification value	188	193	194
Iodine number	154	157	160
Acid number	0.55	64.25	106.48

The results of the analyses of lumbang oil quoted by Wilcox and Thompson and of those of Aguilar vary somewhat, but they all have the same characteristics of high iodine and saponification values.

The constants of Philippine lumbang oil are quite similar to those of tung and linseed oils. This is shown by the work of Richmond and Rosario, the results of which are recorded in Table 18. In view of this similarity, it is not surprising that lumbang oil has properties very similar to those of tung and linseed oils and that it may be used for like purposes.

TABLE 18.—*Constants of lumbang, tung and linseed oils.*

[Data from Richmond and Rosario.]

Constants.	Lumbang (Aleurites moluccana.)	Bagilumbang (Aleurites trisperma.)	Chinese wood or tung oil (Aleurites sp.)	Linseed oil.
Specific gravity at 15° C	0.925-0.927	0.9368	0.9425	0.9368
Acid value (milligrams of potash per one gram of oil)	2.115	2.150	4.547 / 4.568	3.18
Saponification value (milligrams of potash per one gram of oil)	193.5	200.3 / 200.5	189.3	186
Iodine value (Hanus)	150.2	158.5	155.7	179
Maumené value	100	86.2	105	103
Refractive index at 60° C	1.4648	1.483	1.5032	1.4687
Hehner value	95.54	95.79	94.32	94.43
Melting point	-12° C.	2°-4° C.	2° C.	
Solidifying point	-22° C.	-6.5° C.	-7.5° C.	-25° C.

Analyses of the oil cakes, which were obtained on a large scale by expelling the oil from the crushed kernels, are given in Table 19.

168837—9

TABLE 19.—*Analyses of lumbang oil cake.*

Constituents.	Sample.	
	1.a	2.b
Oil	8.8	5.5
Moisture	10.00	10.25
Ash	8.28	
Protein	46.16	47.81
Fiber	1.47	
P2O5	4.39	3.68
K2O	1.95	1.53
Mg & Ca		7.19

a Lewkowitsch, Journal of the Society of Chemical Industry, Volume 20 (1901), page 909.
b Semler, H., Die Tropische Agrikultur, Volume 2, page 515.

Although the oil cake apparently has a high food value it cannot, according to Wilcox and Thompson, be used as cattle food because it has a poisonous effect upon stock. It is a matter of common knowledge that the kernels, either fresh or old, are strongly purgative. The cake left after the oil has been extracted from the kernel is used as a fertilizer, chiefly by the Chinese betel-pepper growers.

Lumbang has been very successfully grown by the Division of Investigation, Bureau of Forestry, at Los Baños. The planting of this species was begun by Forester H. M. Curran. Table 20 gives average rates of growth of large numbers of these trees. For the last few years the trees in the plantations have been rather crowded, and the best trees have made considerably faster rates of growth than the average indicated in the table. The smaller trees should be removed so as to leave more space for the larger ones. The trees which will be left permanently in the plantation have, therefore, shown a faster rate of growth than that given in the table.

TABLE 20.—*Growth of Aleurites moluccana (lumbang) in plantations at Los Baños, Laguna.*

Age.	Diameter.	Height.
Years.	cm.	m.
2		3.58
3	4	4.72
4	8	7.28
5	10	8.13
6	12	10.32
8	15	12.40

Trees on the edge of the plantation have produced considerable quantities of nuts for several years, while those in the main stand have produced comparatively few. Some trees flowered and produced fruit when three years old.

Difficulty has been experienced in germinating the seeds of *Aleurites moluccana*. The seeds are very hard-shelled, and untreated seeds have been known to stay in a seed bed for as long as 38 to 150 days before germination. The most satisfactory method of treatment used was to place the seeds on the ground in a single layer and cover them with dried leaves or kogon grass (*Imperata exaltata*). The grass is then burned.

Immediately after burning and while the seeds are still hot, they are thrown into cold water, which results in the cracking of the hard shells. The results obtained by this kind of treatment showed an average germination of more than 30 per cent. The seeds of lumbang are supposed to retain their vitality for a year or more, but we have very little certain knowledge on this point.

As the seeds of lumbang have very hard shells and germinate slowly, large quantities of them accumulate on the ground under trees. They can, apparently, lie in this condition for a long time without losing much, if any, of their oil content.

The yield of nuts per tree has not been determined accurately, and the common method of gathering the nuts makes such a determination difficult. Some people in Laguna, who engage in the business, estimate the yield from a tree at from 5,000 to 15,000 seeds a year. As the nuts average about 10 grams each, this would be 50 to 150 kilograms per tree. One man said that he had thirty trees in his plantation and that every year he obtained an average of 300 kilograms of husked seeds. This would be about 30 kilograms of unhusked nuts per tree. Aguilar informs us that he obtained from Cavite two sacks of nuts, each sack weighing about 25 kilograms and each of which, according to the collector, was obtained from a single tree. This estimate agrees rather closely with the one just mentioned. According to the above estimates a tree would yield from 5 to 30 kilograms of oil per year.

The fruits are allowed to fall and lie on the ground until that part of the fruit which surrounds the seed has decayed, after which the nuts are collected.

Aleurites moluccana is a large tree reaching a diameter of 80 to 150 centimeters. The younger parts and inflorescences are hairy. The leaves have long petioles. The blades are 10 to 20 centimeters long and are either entire or lobed. The fruit is ovoid, and 5 to 6 centimeters long. It contains one or two hard-shelled seeds. The seed is about 3 centimeters long and 2.5 centimeters broad. It has a hard, rough, ridged shell about 2.5 millimeters thick. This contains a white, oily, fleshy kernel consisting of a very thin embryo surrounded by a large endosperm. This is in turn covered by a thin, white, papery seed coat. This thin seed coat adheres firmly to both the shell and the kernel, so that the kernel is separated from the shell with difficulty.

This species is distributed from Luzon to Mindanao and Palawan, and recently has been planted in great numbers in Cebu.

ALEURITES TRISPERMA Blanco. (Fig. 46).   BAGILUMBÁNG.

Local names: *Bagilumbáng, balukanád* (Laguna); *banukalág, lumbang-banukalád, lumbang-gúbat* (Cavite); *balukanág* (Batangas); *lumbáng* (Oriental Negros, Camarines). Also reported from Rizal, Tayabas and Davao.

BAGILUMBÁNG OIL

As previously mentioned, oil extracted from the nuts of *Aleurites trisperma* has characteristics which are almost indistinguishable from those of Chinese wood oil or tung oil.

According to Heyne * *Aleurites cordata* R. Br., until recently and erroneously believed to be a source of wood oil, occurs in southern Japan. The constants of this oil are remarkably like those of bagilumbang oil from *Aleurites trisperma*.   ‘

The shells of *Aleurites trisperma* are much more easily cracked than those of *Aleurites moluccana*. Moreover, the kernel is not so difficult to separate from the shell because, when the nut is dry, the kernel shrinks somewhat and may be easily removed after the nuts have been cracked. Richmond and del Rosario † found that one kilo of whole nuts contained 357 grams of shells‘ and 643 grams of kernels.

The oil from the nuts of *Aleurites trisperma* deteriorates when the nuts are stored. Moreover, according to Aguilar, the oil deteriorates also if not kept in an hermetically sealed container.

Aguilar says that the yield of oil by expression at 800 kilograms per square centimeter may reach as high as 56 per cent of the weight of the kernels. Oil prepared from fresh nuts is of very good quality and light amber in color. The constants of bagilumbang oil have been determined by Richmond and Ro-

---

* Heyne, K., De Nuttige Planten van Nederlandsch-Indië, (1913).

† Richmond, G. F. and Rosario, M. V. del, Commercial utilization of some Philippine oil-bearing seeds; preliminary paper. Philippine Journal of Science, Volume 2 (1907), pages 439 to 449.

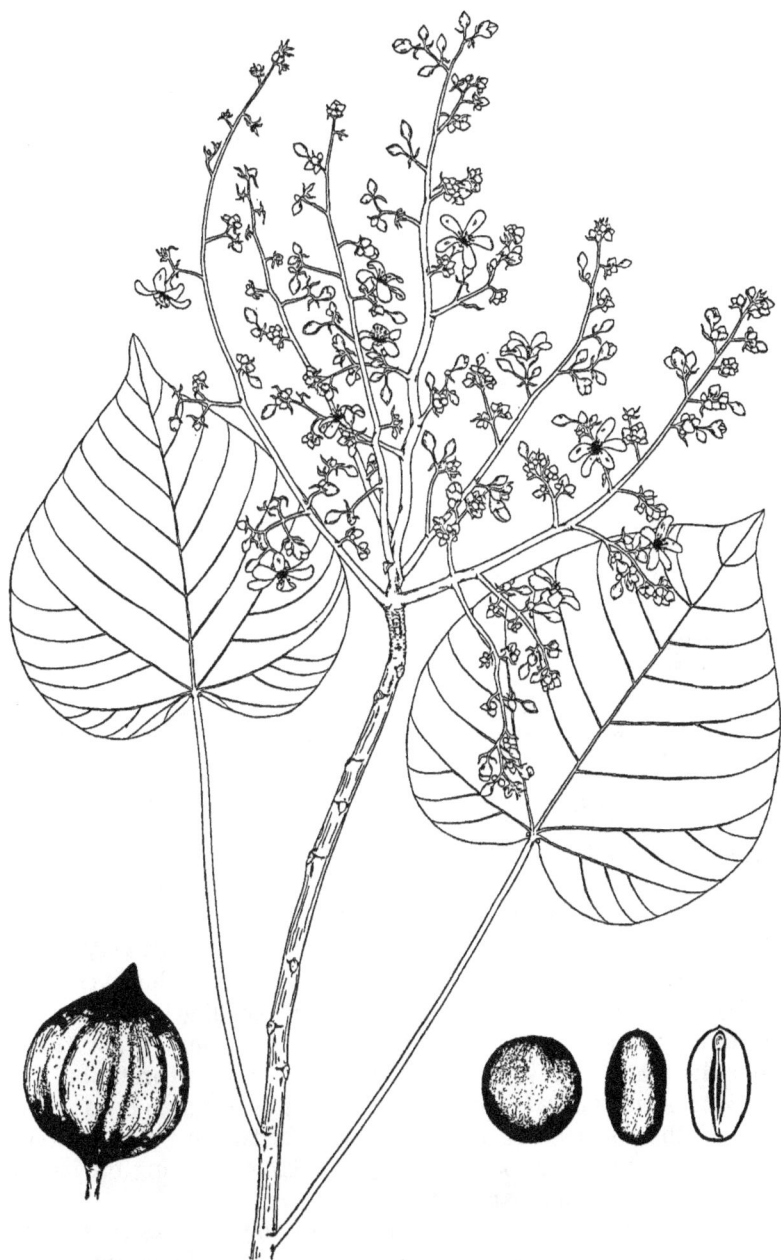

FIGURE 46. ALEURITES TRISPERMA (BAGILUMBANG), THE SOURCE OF BAGILUMBANG
OIL. ×½.

sario. A few of these constants have also been determined by Aguilar. These results are recorded in Table 21. Bagilumbang oil, like lumbang, has high iodine and saponification values and its physical and chemical properties are generally satisfactory. However, when the bagilumbang nuts were kept about sixteen months, they underwent so great a change in the oil value that the yield by expression was reduced from 56 to 40 per cent of the weight of the kernel, and the oil was high in acid value and much darker in color than that obtained from the fresh nuts.

TABLE 21.—*Constants of bagilumbang oil.*

Constants.		Sample.	
		1.a	2.b
Specific gravity {15.0° C		0.9368	
{15.5° C			0.9362
Acid value (milligrams of potash per one gram of oil)		2.150	
Acid value (cc. 0.1 N KOH)			2.22
Saponification value		200.5	191
Iodine value (Hanus)		158.5	166
Maumene value		86.2	
Refractive index (60° C)		1.483	
Hehner value		95.79	
Melting point		2°-4° C.	
Solidifying point		-6.5 C.	

ª Richmond, G. F., and Rosario, M. V. del, Commercial utilization of some Philippine oil-bearing seeds: preliminary paper. Philippine Journal of Science, Volume 2 (1907), page 439.

ᵇ Aguilar, R. H., A comparison of linseed oil and lumbang oils as paint vehicles. Philippine Journal of Science, Volume 12 (1917), page 235.

According to Aguilar, the nuts of *Aleurites trisperma* may be crushed and finely ground in an oil mill and the oil extracted directly from the crushed nuts. However, he found that the oil thus obtained was dirty, highly contaminated with shell particles, dark colored, and had a relatively high acid value. Owing to the small amount of labor involved in shelling the nuts, it seems desirable to extract the oil from the kernels rather than from the whole nuts. It probably would be more profitable to cultivate *Aleurites trisperma* than *Aleurites moluccana*, as the nuts of the former are more easily shelled than those of the latter, and, moreover, bagilumbang oil resembles tung oil more closely than does lumbang oil.

However, *Aleurites trisperma* is not so abundant as *Aleurites moluccana* and consequently the supply of bagilumbang nuts cannot be depended upon until planted trees have begun to bear. The attention of manufacturers should, therefore, be directed for the present to the production of lumbang oil rather than bagilumbang. Although the extraction of oil from bagilumbang nuts alone might not be profitable with the present small supply, it would probably become so if carried on in connection with the extraction of lumbang oil.

The fertilizing value of the cake of *Aleurites trisperma* compares favorably with that of *Aleurites moluccana*, as will be seen from Table 22, taken from Aguilar.

TABLE 22.—*Fertilizing value of bagilumbang* (*Aleurites trisperma*) *cake.*

Constituents.	Cake from kernel.	Cake from crushed nuts.
	Per cent.	*Per cent.*
Moisture	7.67	9.45
Nitrogen (N2)	6.20	2.99
Potash (K2O)	1.79	0.90
Phosphorus (P2O5)	1.13	0.95

Planting experiments carried on by the Division of Investigation, Bureau of Forestry, at Los Baños showed a germination of 98 per cent, germination taking place in nineteen days. At the end of the first year the plants had an average height of 54 centimeters.

This species, like *Aleurites moluccana*, was hardy and grew rapidly. The average rates of growth of large numbers of trees are given in Table 23.

TABLE 23.—*Growth of Aleurites trisperma* (*bagilumbang*) *in plantations at Los Baños, Laguna.*

Age.	Diameter.	Height.
Years.	*cm.*	*m.*
2		1.34
3	5	3.15
5	7	5.08

Aleurites trisperma is a tree 10 to 15 meters or more in height. It does not have hairs except on the inflorescences. The fruit is 5 to 6 centimeters in diameter, somewhat rounded and angled, opens later along the angles, and usually has three cells, each of which contains a single seed. The seed is somewhat circular, flattened, rather smooth, but with numerous small ridges. It has a hard, brittle shell about 0.5 millimeter thick. This contains a white, oily, fleshy kernel consisting of a very thin embryo surrounded by a large endosperm. This in turn is covered by a thin, white, papery seed coat. When dry the kernel with the thin seed coat shrinks slightly away from the shell, so that the shell and kernel are easily separated. The kernels, when fresh, have a pleasant nutty flavor, but leave a burning sensation in mouth, throat, esophagus and stomach; even a part of one nut may cause either violent vomiting within half an hour or else a terrific diarrhœa, beginning within a few hours after eating and lasting from 12 to 24 hours.

This species is a native of the Philippines and is not found outside of the Archipelago. It is apparently not abundant, but quantities sufficient for extensive planting can be secured every year.

Genus CROTON

CROTON TIGLIUM L. (Fig. 47).   CROTON OIL PLANT.

Local names: *Gasi* (Zambales); *kamaisá* (Rizal, Mindoro); *kamausá* (Bulacan); *kaslá* (Balabac Island); *makaslá* (Busuanga Island); *malapi* (Basilan); *marachuite* (Ilocos Sur); *saligau* (Union, Benguet, Cagayan); *túba* (Negros, Camarines, Sorsogon, Samar, Cagayan, Marinduque, Leyte, Rizal, Mindoro, Tayabas); *tubang-makaisá* (Tayabas, Camarines); *tuba-túba* (Negros, Camarines); *tublí* (Lanao).

CROTON OIL

The seeds of this plant yield the croton oil of commerce, which is used chiefly in pharmaceutical preparations. The fruits or crushed leaves of this species are used in poisoning fishes. When the seeds are used for this purpose, they are pulverized and put in sacks which are placed in ponds or rivers.

According to Lewkowitsch,[*] the seeds of *Croton tiglium* yield 53 to 56 per cent of croton oil. The oil has a yellow, orange, or brown color, according to its age. It has a nauseous odor, a burning taste, and acts as a very powerful purgative. It dissolves in petroleum ether in all proportions, differing in this respect from castor oil. It has the following constants (Lewkowitsch):

Specific gravity (15°)	0.9437
Solidifying point	—7°
Saponification value (Mgrms KOH)	192.9–215.6
Iodine value	101.7–109.1
Reichert-Meissl value (CC.1/10 KOH)	12.1–13.56
Refractive index (26°)	1.4781
Oleo-refractometer (22°)	+35°
Butyro-refractometer (27°)	68°–77.5°

Croton tiglium is a shrub or very small tree. The leaves are alternate, usually somewhat rounded at the base, pointed at the tip, with toothed margins, and from 7 to 12 centimeters in length.

---

[*] Lewkowitsch, J., Oils, fats, and waxes (1915).

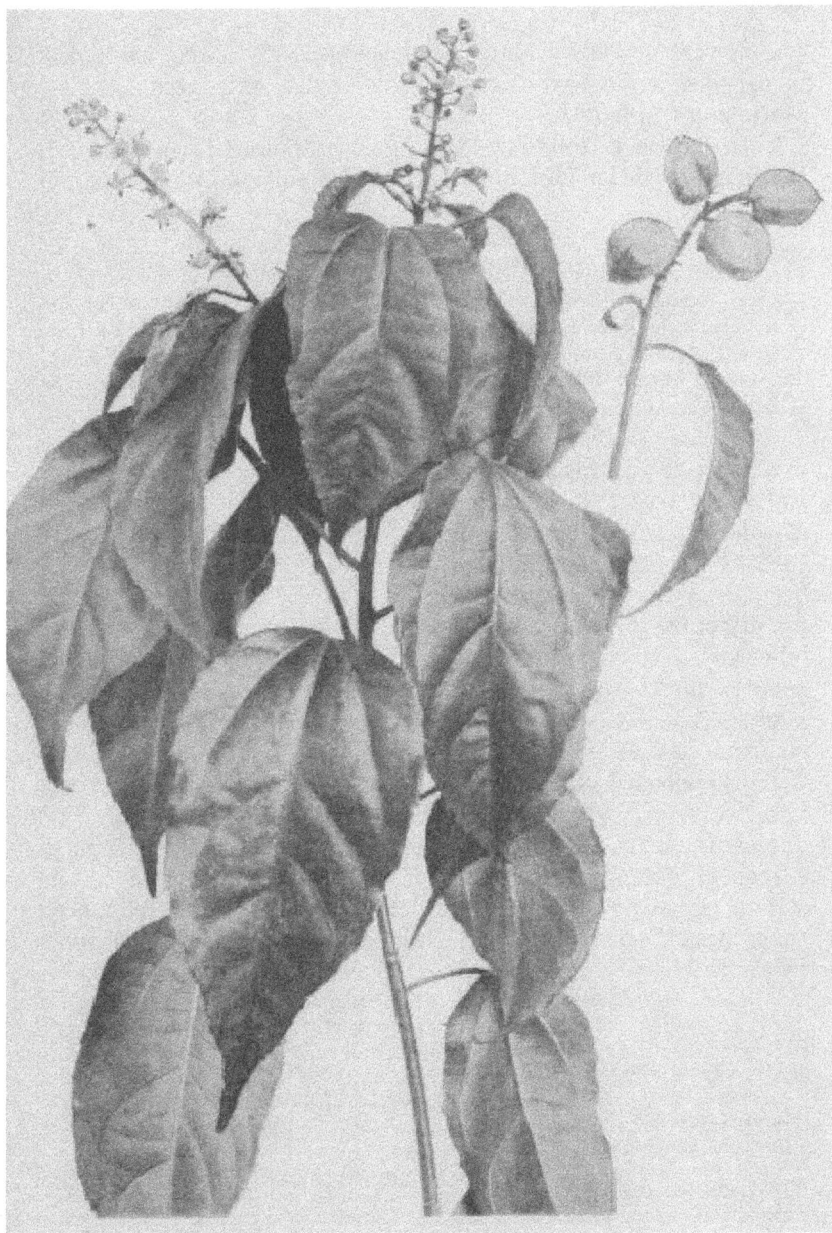

FIGURE 47. CROTON TIGLIUM, THE SOURCE OF CROTON OIL.

The flowers are small and inconspicuous. The seeds are borne
in capsules which are usually three-angled and from 1.5 to 2
centimeters in length.

This species is found wild in the Philippines from northern
Luzon to southern Mindanao. It is also cultivated to a limited
extent.

Genus JATROPHA

JATROPHA CURCAS L. (Fig. 48). TÚBANG-BÁKOD or PHYSIC NUT.

Local names: *Galumbáng* (Pampanga); *kirisól* (Bulacan); *takumbáu*
(Zambales); *tagumbáu* (Ilocos Sur, Pangasinan, Bontoc); *tañgan-táñgan*
(Bataan, Manila); *tañgantáñgan-túba* (Bulacan); *tau-uá* (Ilocos Sur);
taua-tauá (Abra); *túba* (Rizal, Manila, Camarines, Mindoro); *tuba-túba*
(Leyte); *túbang-bákod* (Laguna, Rizal).

PHYSIC-NUT OIL

The seeds of this species furnish an oil used as an emetic
and purgative. The oil has been used for illuminating purposes
in some parts of the Philippines. It is known in commerce as
curcas oil. According to Richmond and Del Rosario * this oil
belongs to the class of semidrying oils and is employed in the
manufacture of soaps and candles and also as an illuminant and
lubricant, but because of its drying properties it is not well
adapted for the last-mentioned purpose. In India it is used as
a purgative. A single fresh seed, eaten raw, may cause both
vomiting and severe diarrhoea.

Lewkowitsch † states that the fresh oil has a pale color, but
becomes yellow with a reddish tint on exposure to the air. Its
unpleasant odor is characteristic, and may serve to distinguish
curcas oil from other oils; it is further characterized by its
strong purgative properties, which are much more pronounced
than those of castor oil. The constants of curcas oil are given
in Table 24.

TABLE 24.—*Constants of physic nut oil.*

Constants.	(a)	(b)	(c)
Acid value	8.5	19	11
Saponification value		192.4	192.6
Unsaponifiable value	0.5		
Acetyl value	8.4		
Reichert-Meissl value		0.5	0.5
Iodine value		89	88

ª Lewkowitsch, J. Oils, fats, and waxes.
ᵇ and ᶜ Heyne, K., De Nuttige Planten van Nederlandsch-Indië (1913).

* Richmond, G. F., and Rosario, M. V. del, Commercial utilization of some
Philippine oil-bearing seeds; preliminary paper. Philippine Journal of
Science, Section A, Volume 2 (1907), page 446.

† Lewkowitsch, J., Oils, fats, and waxes (1915).

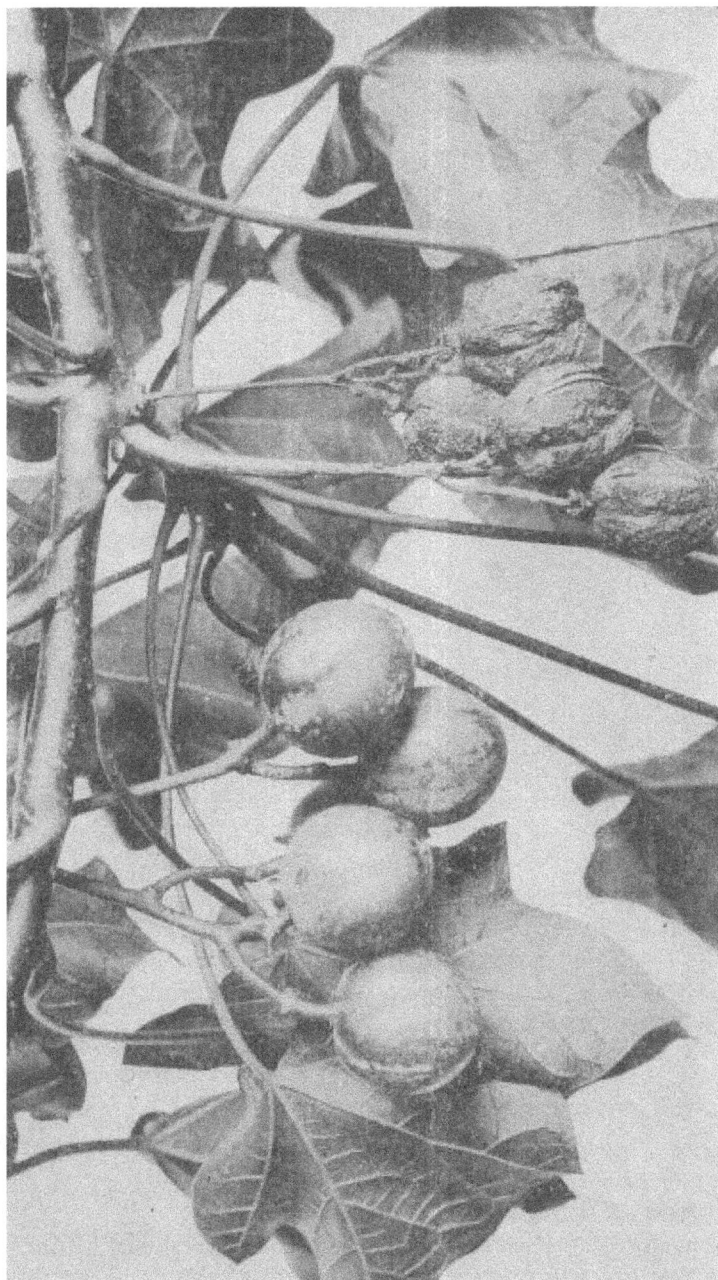

FIGURE 48. JATROPHA CURCAS (TÚBANG-BÁKOD), THE SOURCE OF PHYSIC-NUT OIL.

Richmond and Rosario say that the physic nuts they examined gave 45 per cent of hulls and 55 per cent of kernels; the latter yielded by extraction with chloroform 63.05 per cent of oil, which corresponds to 34.65 per cent calculated on the basis of whole seeds.

Jatropha curcas is an erect shrub or small tree 2 to 5 meters in height. The leaves are entire, angular or somewhat 3- to 5-lobed, and 10 to 18 centimeters long; the apex is pointed, the base heart-shaped, the petiole long. The flowers are greenish white, and 7 to 8 millimeters in diameter. The capsule is rounded, at first fleshy, but later becoming dry, and composed of 2 or 3 one-seeded divisions which are 3 or 4 centimeters long.

This species is a native of tropical America, but is now thoroughly naturalized and widely distributed throughout the Philippines, being most commonly cultivated in towns as a hedge-plant. Hence the name tubang-bakod, *túba* being a name given to many plants of this family used for poisoning fish and *bákod* the Tagalog word for hedge or fence.

JATROPHA MULTIFIDA L.   MANÁ.

Local name: *Maná* (Spanish-Filipino).

MANÁ OIL

According to Heyne * the seeds are poisonous and contain about 30 per cent of oil, which is apparently very similar to that of *Jatropha curcas*. It is used in Java more for illuminating purposes than as a purgative.

Jatropha multifida is a shrub 2 or 3 meters in height. The petioles are as long as the leaves. The leaves are alternate, 15 to 30 centimeters long and divided nearly to the base into about ten rather narrow lobes, which are in turn frequently lobed. The flowers are red and 5 to 6 millimeters long. The capsule is somewhat three-angled and about 2 centimeters long.

This species is occasionally cultivated in the Philippines and is distributed from Luzon to Mindanao.

Genus MALLOTUS

MALLOTUS PHILIPPINENSIS Muell. Arg.   BANÁTO.

BANÁTO OIL

A description and the local names of this species are given in the section on dyes.

According to Watt † the seeds yield 5.83 per cent of a bland

---

* Heyne, K., De Nuttige Planten van Nederlandsch-Indië, Volume 3 (1917), page 100.

† Watt, G., The commercial products of India (1908), page 757.

oil. It is used medicinally by the people of India and many writers recommend it as worthy of investigation.*

Hefter † says that the yield of oil is 20 to 24 per cent.

Genus RICINUS

RICINUS COMMUNIS L. (Fig. 49).   TAÑGAN-TÁÑGAN or CASTOR-OIL. PLANT.

Local names: *Katana* (Batanes Islands); *lansina* (Batangas); *talampúnai* (Laguna); *tañgantáñgan* (Ilocos Norte and Sur, Abra, Cagayan, Pangasinan, Pampanga, Zambales, Bataan, Bulacan, Rizal, Manila, Laguna, Tayabas, Camarines, Albay, Sorsogon, Masbate, Capiz, Misamis, Cuyo Islands); *tau-ua-tau-uá* (Ilocos Norte, Bontoc, Pangasinan).

CASTOR OIL

This plant, the source of the castor oil of commerce, grows wild in all parts of the Philippines, but the seeds are said to be very poor in oil. According to the Bureau of Agriculture, only imported seeds of improved varieties should be planted.

Castor oil is used medicinally as a purgative. It is also used in the manufacture of Turkey-red oils and in making soap. It is employed as a lubricant, as a preservative of leather, and for other purposes. Recently the demand for castor oil has increased owing to the fact that it is used as a lubricant for airplane engines.

Bottler and Sabin ‡ state:

Castor-oil is used as an ingredient for "artificial skin" varnishes, such as one composed of shellac 1 part, alcohol 3 parts, castor-oil ⅛ part; or another, 8 parts collodion to 1 part castor-oil; it is also used in retouching-varnishes and negative varnishes in photography.

To give elasticity to spirit varnishes, it is thinned with alcohol to the consistency of the varnish, and added to it.

Castor oil is colorless or slightly greenish. Commercially it is manufactured by expression or extraction. The best quality, which is used for medicinal purposes, can only be prepared by expression in the cold, as the poisonous alkaloid, ricine, does not pass into the oil under these conditions. The expressed oil cake contains the poisonous alkaloid and is unfit for use as cattle food. It is serviceable, however, as an excellent fertilizer.

Scherubel § discusses the cultivation, harvest, and extraction

---

* Watt, G., Dictionary of the economic products of India, Volume 5 (1891), page 122.

† Hefter, G., Technologie der Fette und Öle (1908).

‡ Bottler, M., and Sabin, A. H., German and American varnish making, page 48.

§ Scherubel, E., Journal of the Department of Agriculture, Victoria, Volume 16 (1918), page 505.

of oil from the castor-oil seeds and states that seeds from two varieties grown wild in Australia contained 47 to 49 per cent of oil. This yield is somewhat less than that obtained from Calcutta and Java seeds, which give about 53 per cent of oil.

The process of refining castor oil consists largely in removing albumen by steaming the oil. The albumen and part of the enzyme which has passed into the oil are thus coagulated and removed by filtering. Castor oil keeps very well when refined properly and does not easily become rancid. The percentage of free fatty acids does not increase considerably on standing. According to Lewkowitsch * a sample exposed to the athmosphere for four years contained only 1 per cent of free fatty acids.

Castor oil has the following constants (Lewkowitsch):

Specific gravity (15.5°), 0.9591.
Solidifying point –10° to –12°.
Saponification value (Mgrms KOH) 176.7 to 186.6.
Iodine value 81.4 to 90.6.
Reichert-Meissl value (C.C.1/10 norm. KOH) 1.1.
Acetyl value 149.9 to 150.5.
Maumené test 46° to 47°.
Refractive index (15°) 1.4795 to 1.4803.
Oleo-refractometer (22°) 37 to 46.
Butyro-refractometer (25°) 78°.
Viscosity (Redwood's viscosimeter) 1160 to 1190.

As shown by the figures above, the acetyl value is unusually high. Mitchell † states that castor oil has an acetyl value of about 150 and emphasizes the fact that other oils and fats have acetyl values ranging from about 2 (coconut oil) to 15 (cottonseed oil) and 19 (croton oil).

According to Richmond and Rosario ‡ castor oil could be manufactured in a coconut-oil mill and, if the plant were cultivated on a sufficient scale, there would be a possibility of the commercial production of this oil for lubricating and illuminating purposes. It could probably be sold as cheaply as coconut oil, which is now used extensively in food products.

Ricinus communis is a coarse, erect, somewhat woody bush about 1 to 4 meters high. The leaves are smooth, alternate, 20 to 60 centimeters in diameter and palmately divided, with pointed lobes. The leaves and stems are green or purplish. The fruit

---

* Lewkowitsch, J., oils, fats, and waxes, (1915).
† Mitchell, C. A., Edible oils and fats, (1918).
‡ Richmond, G. F., and Rosario, M. V. del, Commercial utilization of some Philippine oil-bearing seeds: preliminary paper. Philippine Journal of Science, Section A, Volume 2 (1907), page 448.

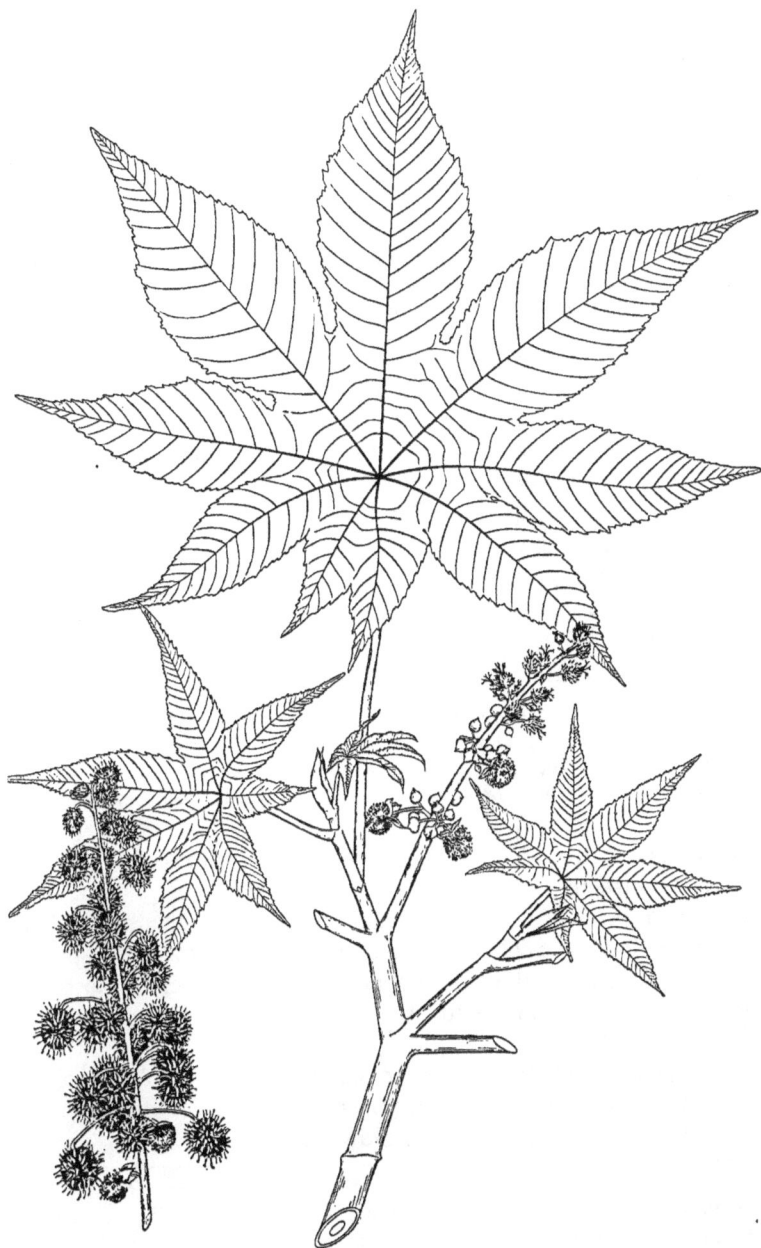

FIGURE 49. RICINUS COMMUNIS (TANGAN-TANGAN), THE SOURCE OF CASTOR OIL.
X½.

is an ovoid capsule, 1 to 1.5 centimeters long, and covered with soft, spine-like processes.

Family ANACARDIACEAE

Genus ANACARDIUM

ANACARDIUM OCCIDENTALE L.   KASÚI or CASHEW NUT.

Local names: *Balúbad* or *balúbar* (Bataan, Pampanga, Bulacan); *balúbat* (Bataan, Mindoro); *batúban* (Bataan); *balúbog* (Bulacan); *kachúi* (Palawan); *kasói* or *kasúi* (Isabela, Ilocos Norte and Sur, Abra, Tarlac, Bataan, Zambales, Manila, Rizal, Laguna, Batangas, Camarines, Mindoro, Capiz, Marinduque, Palawan, Misamis, Cuyo Islands, Zamboanga); *kosíng* (Amburayan); *sambalduke* (Pangasinan).

CASHEW-NUT OIL

The roasted kernels are often used to make a very savory nut candy, and also, according to Richmond and Rosario,* for the adulteration of chocolate. They say that the expressed kernels yield a sweet, yellowish oil.

Lewkowitsch † states that the yield of oil from the kernels is 47.2 per cent and that the oil has the following constants:

Saponification value	195
Iodine value	84
Refractive index (20°)	1.4702

Watt ‡ says that:

* * * Two oils are obtainable from this plant: (1) a light-yellow from the pressed kernels, of which the finest quality is equal to almond oil; and (2) "Cardole," obtained from the shell of the nut—an acrid and powerful fluid efficacious for preserving carved wood, books, etc., against white ants. * * *

Watt also mentions that the bark yields a gum which is obnoxious to insects.

Anacardium occidentale is a small tree with a trunk which is usually small and crooked. It has a large, yellow, pear-shaped fruit, with a kidney-shaped seed attached to one end. Both the fruit and seed are edible, the fruit raw and the kernels raw or roasted.

This species, introduced at an early date from America, is widely distributed in the Philippines. It is cultivated in towns and on farms, and runs wild in old clearings.

---

* Richmond, G. F., and Rosario, M. V. del, Commercial utilization of some Philippine oil-bearing seeds; preliminary paper. Philippine Journal of Science, Section A, Volume 2 (1907), page 445.

† Lewkowitsch, J., Oils, fats, and waxes (1915).

‡ Watt, George, The commercial products of India (1908).

Family CELASTRACEAE

Genus CELASTRUS

CELASTRUS PANICULATA Willd.

CELASTRUS PANICULATA OIL

According to Watt: *

The seeds yield by expression a deep scarlet or yellow oil, used medicinally. The oil deposits a quantity of fat after it has been kept a short time. Its odour is pungent and acrid, and treated with sulphuric acid it turns of a dark bistre colour. It is much admired as an external application along with a poultice of the crushed seeds. It is also burnt in lamps, and employed in certain religious ceremonies. The seeds submitted to destructive distillation yield the "Oleum Nigrum," an empyreumatic black oily fluid employed medicinally in the treatment of *beri-beri* (*Cooke*). According to Dr. Dymock, the seeds are distilled along with benzoin, cloves, nutmegs, and mace. This oil is manufactured in the Northern Circars, the best in Vizagapatam and Ellore, where it is sold in small blue or black bottles, each containing about ¼ oz., at prices from 12 annas to one rupee a bottle.

Lewkowitsch † states that:

The seeds from the shrub *Celastrus paniculatus* yield a dark-red pungent oil from which "stearine" separates on standing. In Ceylon this oil is known as "Duhudu oil," and serves as a nerve stimulant; it is also used there for external application to sores.

Celastrus paniculata is a large, woody vine. The leaves are alternate, somewhat oval shaped, pointed at the tip, rounded or slightly pointed at the base, with toothed margins, and 5 to 12 centimeters long. The inflorescences are 7 to 18 centimeters long. The flowers are numerous, greenish or greenish white, and about .5 millimeter in diameter. The fruit is an ovoid or somewhat rounded, yellow capsule which is 7 to 9 centimeters long and three-celled.

This species is distributed from northern Luzon to Mindanao and Palawan.

Family SAPINDACEAE

Genus GANOPHYLLUM

GANOPHYLLUM FALCATUM Blume. (Fig. 50). ARÁÑGEN.

Local names: *Aráñgen* (Iloko in Union, Pangasinan); *bagusalai* (Misamis); *gogong-láñgil* (Cavite); *gogolíñgin* (Pampanga); *gúgo* (Tablas Island); *hálas* (Capiz); *malatumbága* (Bataan); *odó* (Mindoro); *palumpúng, pararan* (Davao); *sáleng* (Bontoc); *tugábi* (Tayabas).

---

* Watt, G., A dictionary of the economic products of India, Volume 2 (1889), page 238.

† Lewkowitsch, J., Oils, fats, and waxes, Volume 2 (1915), page 338.

ARÁÑGEN OIL

The seeds of this species yield a solid fat used for illumination. The people of the hills back of San Fernando, La Union, chiefly the Igorotes, have extracted this product for many years. The seeds are crushed and then boiled, when the oil floats on the surface. Wells,* who examined this product, says that even with potash it makes a good hard soap.

Ganophyllum falcatum is a tree reaching a height of about 25 meters and a diameter of about 70 centimeters. The leaves are alternate, 20 to 35 centimeters long, and pinnate with alternate leaflets which are inequilateral, pointed at the tip, oblique at the base, and from 5 to 12 centimeters in length. The flowers are small, yellowish, and occur in large numbers on compound flowering shoots. The fruits are about 1.5 centimeters in length, pointed at the tip, rounded at the base, and contain a single seed. The wood is hard and heavy, of fine texture, yellowish white, apparently durable, and is used locally for posts and other structural parts of houses.

This species is distributed from northern Luzon to Mindanao.

Genus **NEPHELIUM**

NEPHELIUM LAPPACEUM L.   Usáu or Rambután.

RAMBUTÁN TALLOW

A description, figure, and the local names of this species are given in the bulletin on edible plants.

Hefter † states that the seeds of *Nephelium lappaceum* yield 40 to 48 per cent of rambután tallow.

According to Baczewski ‡ this tallow has the following constants:

Specific gravity	0.9236
Solidifying point	38°-39°
Melting point	42°-46°
Saponification value	193.8
Iodine value	39.4

The insoluble fatty acids of this tallow contain 45.5 per cent of oleic acid.

---

* Wells, A. H., Chief, Division of Organic Chemistry, Bureau of Science, Manila.

† Hefter, G., Technologie der Fette und Öle, Volume 2 (1908), page 652.

‡ Baczewski, M., Chemische untersuchung der Samen von Nephelium lappaceum und des darin enthaltenen fettes. Monatshefte für Chemie, ‹ Volume 16 (1895), page 866.

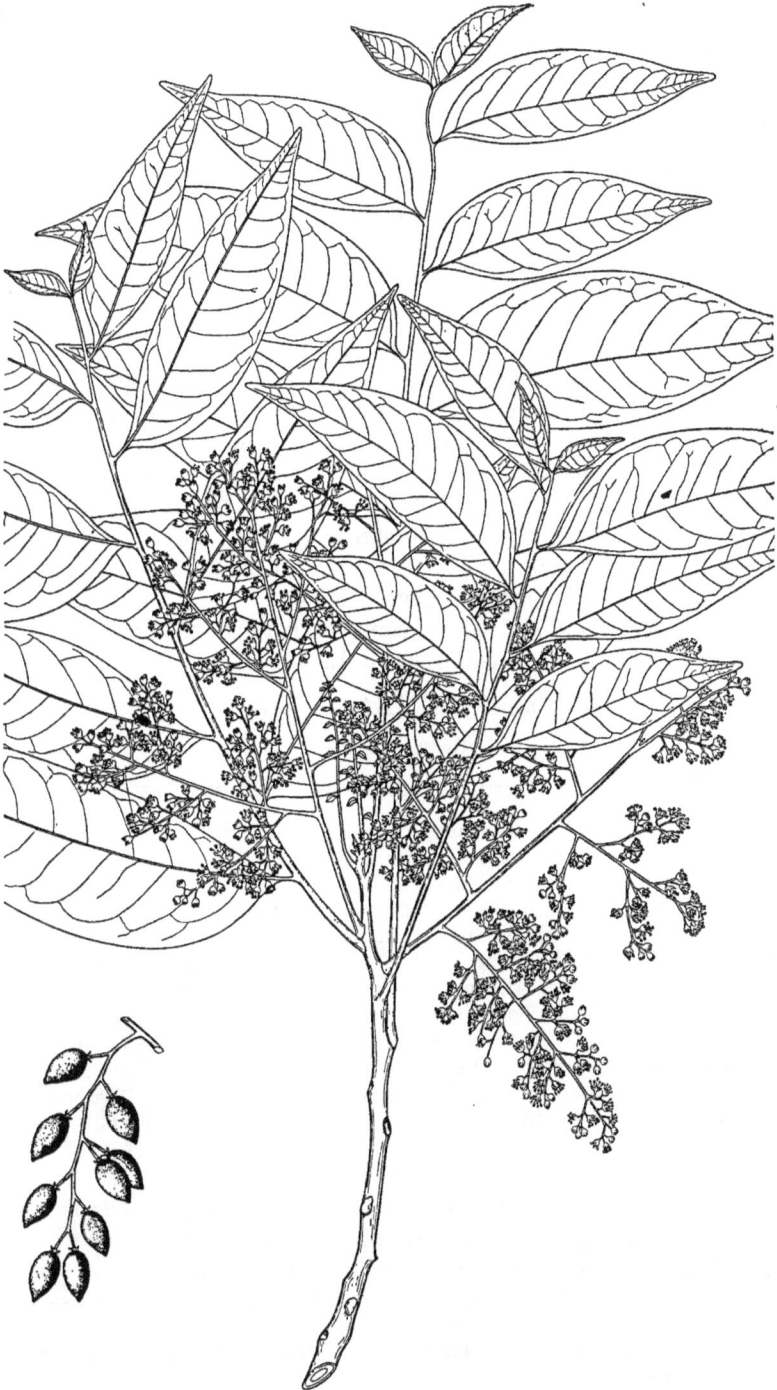

FIGURE 50. GANOPHYLLUM FALCATUM (ARANGEN). X⅓.

NEPHELIUM MUTABILE Blanco.   BULÁLA.

Local names: *Alpái* (Laguna); *bakaláu* (Pangasinan); *balimbíñgan* (Lanao); *bulála* (Camarines, Tayabas, Laguna, Rizal); *kakao-kakao* (Surigao); *karayo* (Mindoro); *laguan* (Tayabas); *malamputian* (Samar); *maráñgis* (Cagayan); *pangyáu* (Rizal).

BULÁLA OIL

Heyne * reports that according to Greshoff the seeds contain 29.2 per cent of fat melting at 34° C. He says that it was formerly used as a lamp oil.

Nephelium mutabile is a tree reaching a height of about 25 meters and a diameter of 45 centimeters. The leaves are alternate and compound, with rather large, smooth, alternate leaflets, which are pointed at both ends. The flowers are small and occur in considerable numbers on simple or compound inflorescences. The fruits are red, about 4 centimeters in length, and completely covered with numerous, rather soft projections. The flesh is white, abundant, juicy, and of very good flavor. It surrounds a single, rather large seed.

This species is distributed from northern Luzon to southern Mindanao and is very common in Luzon.

Family BOMBACACEAE

Genus CEIBA

CEIBA PENTANDRA Gaertn. (Fig. 51).   COTTON TREE or KÁPOK.

Local names: *Balios* (Bulacan); *basanglái* (Ilocos Sur, Abra); *bobói*, *bubúi* (Bulacan, Bataan, Cavite, Batangas, Rizal, Laguna, Tayabas, Mindoro); *boibói* (Capiz); *búlak* (Abra, Zambales, Pampanga, Bulacan, Cavite); *búlak-dondól* (Cebu); *búlak-kastíla* (Pampanga); *búlak-sino* (Bulacan, Bataan, Cavite, Batangas, Rizal, Laguna, Tayabas, Mindoro); *dogdól* (Cebu); *doldól* (Leyte, Samar, Iloilo, Antique, Capiz, Bohol, Cebu, Cuyo Islands); *dondól* (Cebu); *gápas* (Misamis); *kápah* (Zambales); *kápak* (Bulacan, Rizal, Bohol); *kápas* (Ilocos Norte and Sur, Zambales); *kápas-sanglái* (Ilocos Norte and Sur, Abra); *kápok* or *kapók* (Tarlac, Sorsogon, Masbate, Davao and other parts of Mindanao, Basilan, Sulu group); *kapös* (Pangasinan); *kasanglái* (Pangasinan); *káyo* (Camarines, Albay, Sorsogon, Samar, Leyte, Capiz, Antique, Iloilo, Cebu, Bohol); *sanglái* (Abra).

KÁPOK OIL

An oil resembling cotton-seed oil is extracted from the kapok seeds. It has a greenish-yellow color and a taste and odor which is not unpleasant. The oil is used for the manufacture of soap and as a substitute for cotton-seed oil. Concerning the use of

---

* Heyne, K., De Nuttige Planten van Nederlandsch-Indië, Volume 3 (1917), page 162.

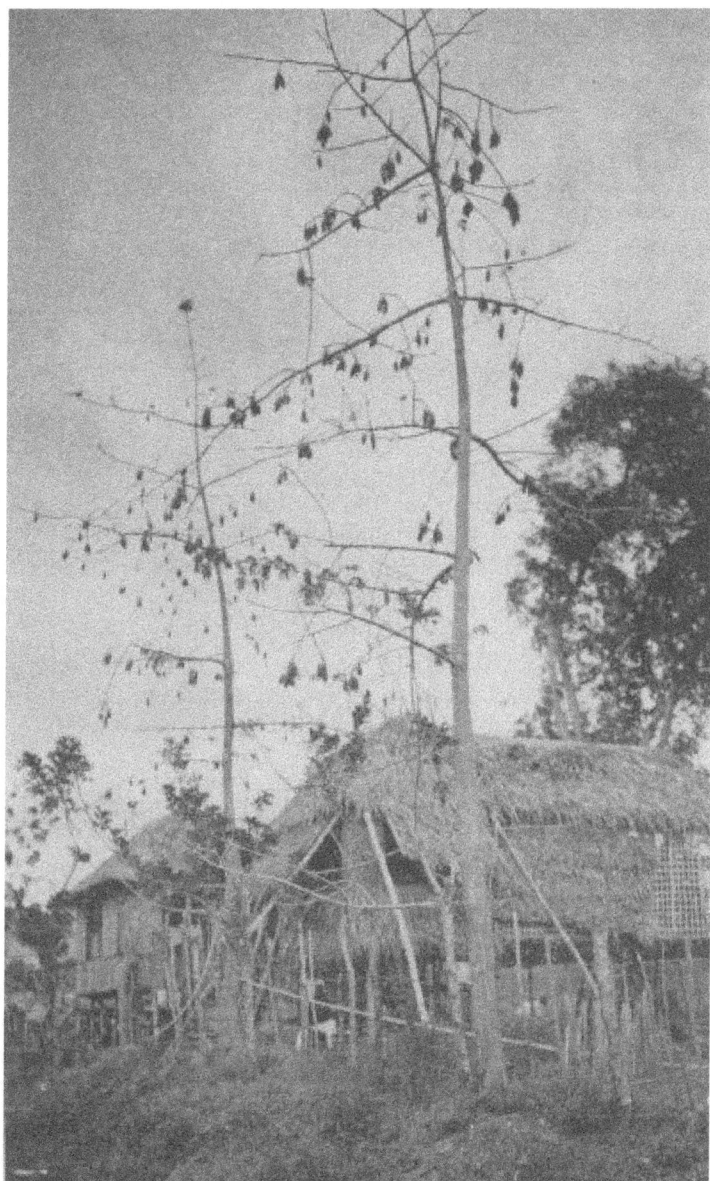

FIGURE 51. CEIBA PENTANDRA (KAPOK), THE SOURCE OF KAPOK OIL.

kapok oil in Marseilles for soap making, the American Perfumer * states:

* * * The seed is treated in two mills, both of which are chiefly devoted to the crushing of other seeds. Only one pressing is the rule, although in some cases hot water is poured over the residue, which is then pressed again. The oil is then filtered, but it requires neither bleaching, deodorizing, nor any other treatment. In the Marseilles mills the average yield in oil from this seed is about 15 per cent. The price of the oil follows closely that of industrial peanut oil. It takes about 16½ pounds of kapok to make a gallon of oil.

Lewkowitsch † says the seeds have the following average composition:

	Per cent.
Oil	24.20
Water	11.85
Ash	5.22
Crude fiber	23.91
Albuminoids	18.92
Carbohydrates, etc	15.90

Experiments carried out by the Philippine Bureau of Agriculture indicate that the fresh cake is valuable as stock food. According to Richmond and del Rosario ‡ the product much resembles ground linseed in food value.

Kapok oil has the following constants (Lewkowitsch): †

Specific gravity at 15° C	0.9235
Solidifying point	29.6°
Saponification value (Mgrms KOH)	181–205
Iodine value	117.9
Maumené test	95
Refractive index	51.3

The oil consists of a mixture of fatty acids, about 70 per cent of which is liquid, while 30 per cent is palmitic acid, which is a solid.

Ceiba pentandra is a slender tree 15 meters or less in height. The trunk is armed with large, scattered spines. The branches are borne in horizontal whorls which are very characteristic. The capsules are about 15 centimeters long, and 5 centimeters thick. They contain black seeds imbedded in fine, silky hairs.

---

* The American Perfumer, Volume 10 (1915–1916), page 298.

† Lewkowitsch, J., Oils, fats, and waxes (1915).

‡ Richmond, G. F. and Rosario, M. V. del, Commercial utilization of some Philippine oil-bearing seeds: preliminary paper. Philippine Journal of Science, Volume 2 (1907), page 445.

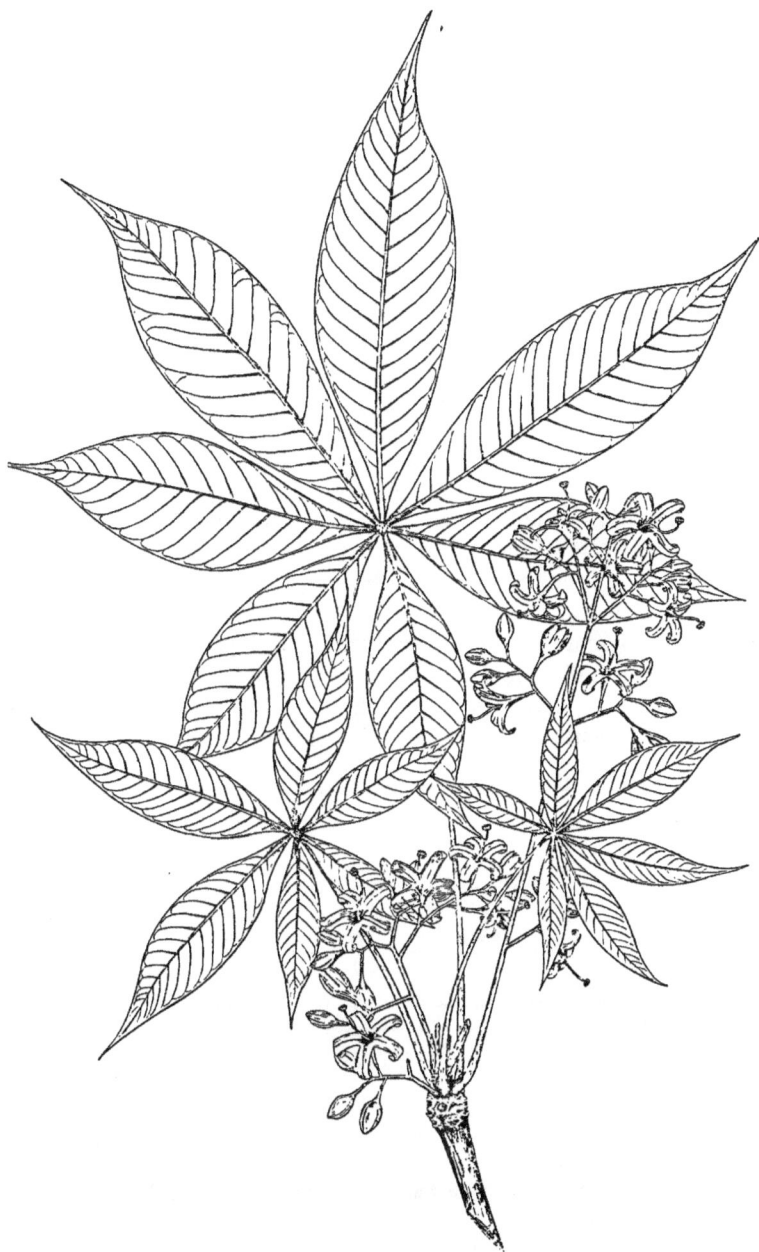

FIGURE 52. STERCULIA FOETIDA (KALUMPÁNG), THE SOURCE OF KALUMPÁNG OIL
X⅓.

The fibers surrounding the seeds are soft, elastic, and immune to moths, and therefore very suitable for stuffing pillows, mattresses, etc., for which purposes they are extensively employed. This species is commonly cultivated, particularly along the highways and in towns, in all parts of the Philippines.

Family STERCULIACEAE

Genus STERCULIA

STERCULIA FOETIDA L. (Figs. 52, 53).   KALUMPÁNG.

Local names: *Bañgár* (Abra); *bañgát, bubúr* (Ilocos Sur); *bobóg* (Iloilo, Palawan); *buñgóg* (Cagayan); *kalumpáng* (Nueva Ecija, Tayabas, Pampanga, Rizal, Bataan, Manila, Laguna, Camarines, Iloilo, Mindoro, Palawan, Cotabato, Apo Island); *kurumpáng* (Davao).

KALUMPÁNG OIL

The fruits of this species and of several others of the genus contain a number of peanut-like, oily kernels. They are more or less laxative when eaten raw. An oil extracted from them is used locally for illuminating purposes. In some parts of the Islands the oil mixed with white earth is utilized as a paint. The oil is a bland, sweet, yellow oil, having a rather high melting point. Brill and Agcaoili * analyzed the dry, shelled seeds and determined the chemical constants of the oil obtained from them. The results are given in Tables 25 and 26. These tables also include the results obtained by Bolton and Jesson.†

TABLE 25.—*Composition of dry, shelled, kalumpang seeds.*

Constituents.	Analysis by	
	Bureau of Science.	Bolton and Jesson.
	Per cent.	*Per cent.*
Fat (by extraction of dry seeds)	51.78	52.0
Protein (N x 6.25)	21.61	
Starch	12.10	
Sugars	5.00	
Cellulose, etc. (by difference)	5.51	
Ash	3.90	

* Brill, H. C., and Agcaoili, F., Philippine oil-bearing seeds and their properties: II. Philippine Journal of Science, Section A, Volume 10 (1915), page 108.

† Analyst, Volume 40 (1915), page 3.

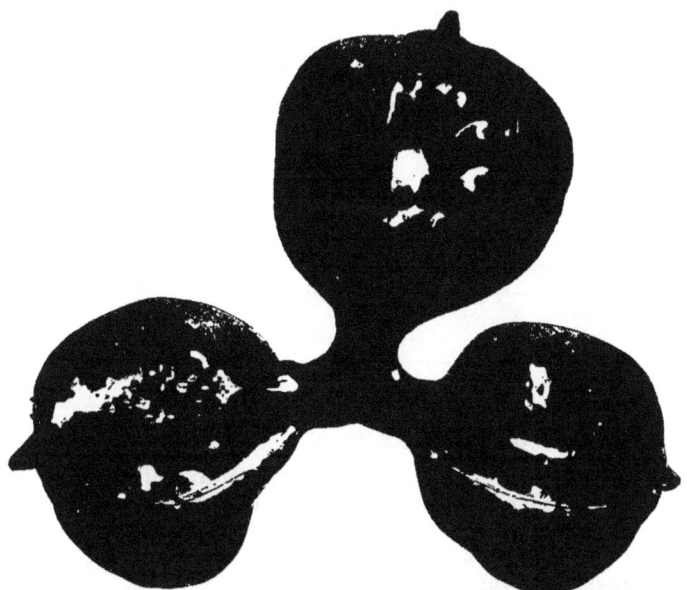

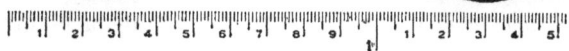

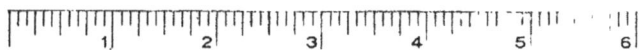

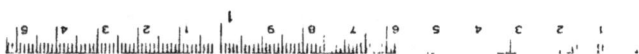

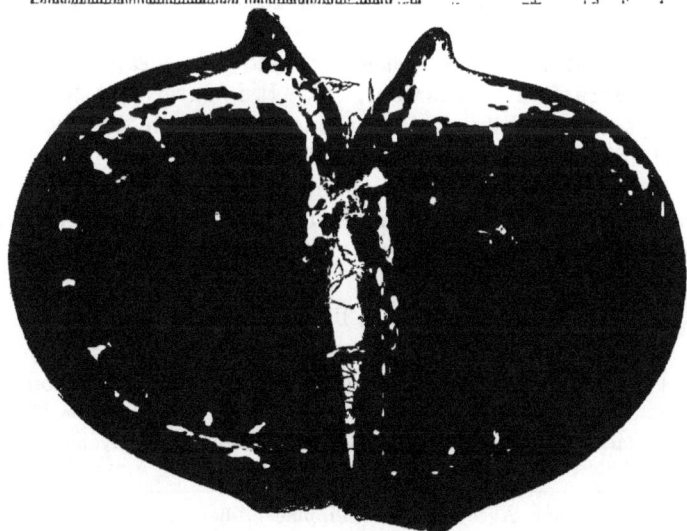

FIGURE 53. FRUITS OF STERCULIA FOETIDA (KALUMPANG), THE SOURCE OF KALUM-PANG OIL.

TABLE 26.—*Chemical constants of kalumpang oil.*

Constants.	Analysis by	
	Bureau of Science.	Bolton and Jesson.
Specific gravity at 30°C	0. 9254	....
Butyro refractometer reading at 40°C	63. 64	....
Iodine value (Hanus)	76. 04	75. 8
Reichert-Meissl value	2. 10	....
Saponification number	212. 01	193. 8
Free fatty acids (oleic) ___per cent__	0. 45	1. 0
Acid value ___cc. N/10 KOH__	0. 30	....

According to Professor DuMez: *

The oil appears to resemble olive oil very much in its physiological action. Administered to dogs in doses of 1.5 to 3 cubic centimeters per kilogram body weight, it acts as a mild laxative. It is nontoxic and has no irritating action. It can be used in the same manner as olive oil and should be especially useful for culinary purposes.

Sterculia foetida is a spreading tree reaching a height of 20 meters or more. The leaves are crowded at the ends of the branches. They are compound, having seven to nine leaflets borne in a whorl at the end of the petiole. The leaflets are 12 to 18 centimeters long. The flowers are rank-smelling, dull yellowish or purplish, and 2 to 2.5 centimeters in diameter. The fruit is large, woody, red, nearly smooth, ovoid, and about 10 centimeters long. It contains 10 to 15 seeds, which are about 2 centimeters long.

The wood of *Sterculia foetida* is used for cheap and temporary construction, box-lumber, etc. It is rarely cut for lumber except occasionally by larger operators, with the cheapest grade of miscellaneous lumber. The wood is soft to very soft and light to very light. The durability is very poor.

This species is found throughout the Philippines, and is distributed from eastern Africa to India through Malaya to northern Australia.

Family GUTTIFERAE

Genus CALOPHYLLUM

CALOPHYLLUM INOPHYLLUM L. (Fig. 54).   BITÁOG or PALOMARIA DE LA PLAYA.

Local names: *Batárau* (Cagayan, Batanes); *bitáog* (Babuyanes, Abra, Union, Zambales, Ilocos Norte and Sur, Bataan, Leyte, Agusan); *bitáoi*

---

* Brill, H. C., and Agcaoili, F., Philippine oil-bearing seeds and their properties: II. Philippine Journal of Science, Section A, Volume 10 (1915), page 109.

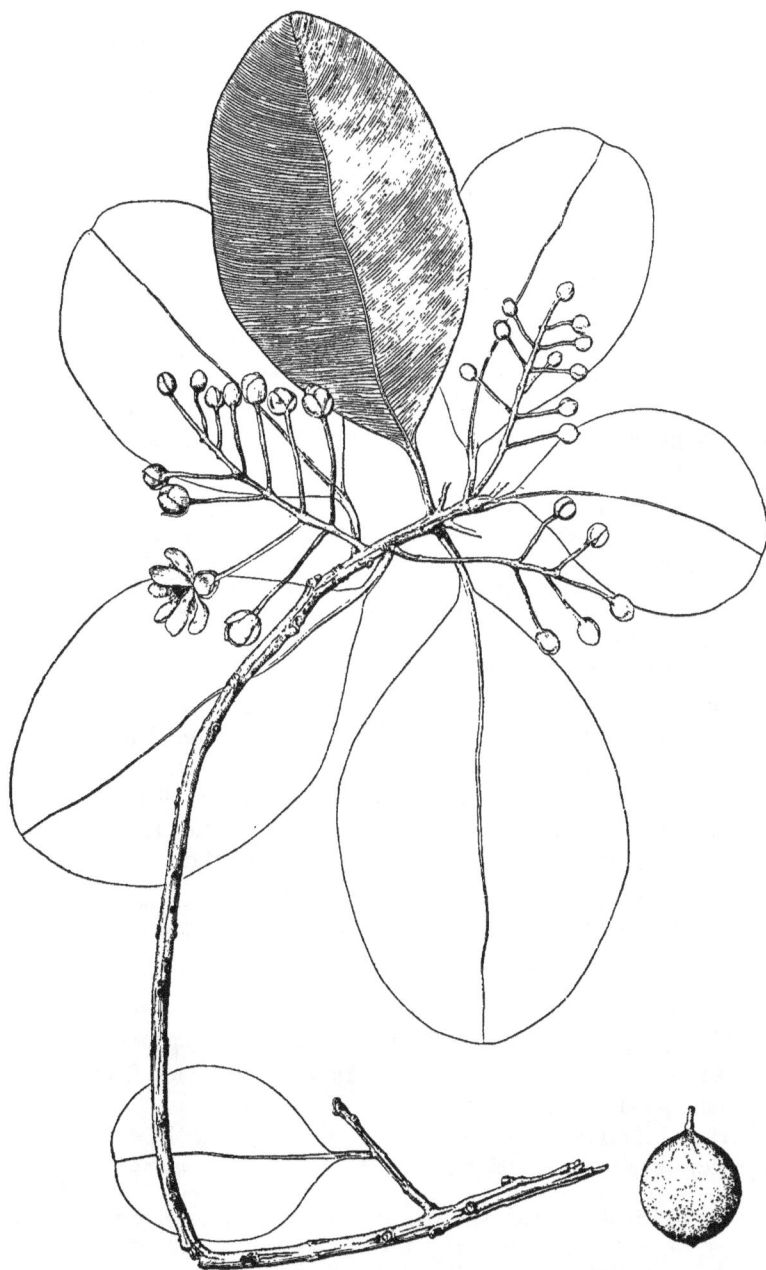

J.Vitan del.

FIGURE 54. CALOPHYLLUM INOPHYLLUM (BITÁOG OR PALOMARIA DE LA PLAYA), THE
SOURCE OF PALOMARIA OIL.

(Pangasinan); *bitóng* (Bataan); *bit-táog* (Cagayan, Camiguin, Isabela); *bittóg* (Bataan); *butálau* (Batangas); *dagkálan* (Isabela); *dangkálan* (Bataan, Tayabas, Camarines, Albay, Mindoro, Masbate, Negros, Capiz, Lanao, Zamboanga, Burias Island, Butuan, Cotabato, Palawan); *dangkáan* (Davao); *palomaría* (Mindoro, Tayabas, Bataan, Zambales, Pangasinan, Nueva Ecija, Cagayan, Manila, Cebu, Zamboanga); *palomaria de la playa* (Bataan, Laguna, Camarines, Mindoro, Misamis, Zamboanga, Basilan); *pamittaógen* (Palaui Island); *tambo-tambo* (Jolo); *vutálau* (Batanes).

BITÁOG OIL

The seeds yield bitáog oil which is greenish-yellow in color and which in some districts is used as an illuminant. Each tree yields several bushels of nuts per year. According to Richmond and del Rosario * 70 to 75 per cent of this oil can be extracted from the kernels. They say that the oil is called domba and in Indo-English, improperly, laurel-nut oil. Concerning its uses they write:

* * * The oil is not serviceable as an edible fat, since it contains a poisonous resin to which the color and odor are due. On the other hand, it finds application as a natural remedy in skin diseases and rheumatism, and it is used for that purpose in many districts of India; it is exported in considerable amounts from Travancore, particularly from Burma, and under the name of "udiloöl" it has been experimentated with in Europe for some time in the treatment of rheumatism.

The oil is said to be excellent for making soap.

G. Fenler † investigated the oil obtained from the nuts of *Calophyllum inophyllum* and states that it is greenish-yellow in color, has a bitter, pungent taste, and is soluble in all proportions in the usual solvents, but is insoluble in absolute alcohol. An examination of the oil gave the following constants:

Specific gravity at 15° C	0.942
Reichert-Meissl number	.13
Acid value	28.45
Saponification value	196
Iodine value	92.8

When heated with caustic soda the oil yields a greenish resin of semiliquid consistency, soluble in alcohol. The fatty acids consist largely of palmitic, oleic, and stearic acid.

Crevost ‡ states that Lefeuvre, by neutralizing the oil of *Calophyllum inophyllum* with caustic potash and separating the soaps

---

* Richmond, G. F., and Rosario, M. V. del, Commercial utilization of some Philippine oil-bearing seeds: preliminary paper. Philippine Journal of Science, Section A, Volume 2 (1907), page 444.

† Chemiker Zeitschrift, Volume 29 (1905), page 15.

‡ Crevost, Ch., Bulletin Economique de l'Indochine, New Series, Volume 8 (1906), page 394.

'thus formed from the remaining oil, found that bitáog oil contains 71.55 per cent of fatty oil and 28.45 per cent of resin. The resin is dark brown in color and melts at 30° to 35°. It is soluble in benzine, carbon disulphide, petroleum ether, alcohol, and other organic solvents. The resin had an iodine value of 125.2 and the acid number (milligrams of caustic potash required to neutralize one gram of resin) was 180.8.

Since bitáog oil consists of a resin dissolved in a neutral oil, it is really a natural varnish and may be useful in the varnish industry.

Watt * says that the nuts are collected twice a year in India, and that they yield 60 per cent of oil.

The seeds of other species of *Calophyllum*, especially *Calophyllum blancoi* Pl. and Tr., also yield an oil used for illuminating purposes.

Calophyllum inophyllum has been grown sucessfully in plantations at Los Baños. In most cases the seeds showed fairly high percentages of germination. The average rates of growth of considerable numbers of trees are given in Table 27.

TABLE 27.—*Growth of Calophyllum inophyllum (bitaog) in plantations at Los Baños, Laguna.*

Age.	Diameter.	Height.
Years.	*cm.*	*m.*
2		.88
3		1.45
4	2	1.93
5	3	3.35
7	4	4.39

According to Crevost † the growth of this species seems to be very rapid, and at the end of two years some seedlings begin to produce fruits. He says that in less than four or five years one can hardly count on anything like a normal, annual production which would perhaps be about 20 to 40 kilos according to the age of the tree. Several highways in Cochinchina and Annam are entirely bordered with this species.

Calophyllum inophyllum is usually a medium-sized or large tree with a very short bole and dense, wide-spreading crown. It occurs on sandy beaches throughout the Islands. The bark

---

* Watt, George, The commercial products of India, (1908).

† Crevost, Ch., Bulletin Economique de l'Indochine, New Series, Volume 8 (1906), page 392.

is 12 to 20 millimeters thick, brown, with a decided yellow tinge, and has a tendency to divide into distinct ridges, which are often broken into irregular rectangular patches by cross fissures. The inner bark is pink to yellowish, with concentric lines of darker color. When the bark is cut, a sticky, yellowish sap exudes. The fruit is the size of a walnut. It has an outer fleshy portion and contains a thin-shelled seed with a hard, oily kernel.

This species is probably distributed in all parts of the Philippines bordering on the coast.

Family DIPTEROCARPACEAE

A fat known as Borneo tallow is obtained from certain dipterocarp trees, especially *Shorea, Hopea*, and *Isoptera*. Hefter * states that Borneo tallow is used in the Sunda Islands as food and for making soap. He says that it has a light green or yellow color and, when in a fresh condition, a pleasant taste, somewhat like that of coco butter.

According to Foxworthy,† this fat is used for manufacturing candles, for cooking purposes, and for lubricating machinery. He further says that it is derived chiefly from *Shorea* and *Isoptera*, and that the seeds of these species have a local value in Borneo of 7.50 dollars per picul.

Two species which Hefter says yield this product, *Shorea balangeran* (Korth.) Dyer and *Isoptera borneensis* Scheff., have been reported from the Philippines.

A tree that is called *Shorea balangeran* (gisok) is distributed in the Philippines from Luzon to Mindanao, but has never been collected in fruit. Foxworthy ‡ says:

Our material credited to this species resembles very closely that shown ₁ in Korthals' original figure [Verh. Nat. Gesch. Bot. (1848) *t. 7*] in leaf and flower characters, except that there are more than fifteen stamens, in some cases about thirty, and the appendage to the connective is ciliate. The style is also shorter than that shown in the figure. I have not seen the type of *Shorea balangeran* and thus do not feel that it is desirable to describe our form as a new species. Much of our material is sterile. The fruit has not yet been collected.

The only records we have of the occurrence of *Isoptera borneensis* in the Philippines are seven collections from the District of Zamboanga, Mindanao, and from Camarines.

---

* Hefter, G., Technologie der Fette und Öle, Volume 2 (1908), page 680.

† Foxworthy, F. W., Minor forest products and jungle produce. British North Borneo Bulletin No. 1 (1916), page 57.

‡ Foxworthy, F. W., Philippine Dipterocarpaceae, II. Philippine Journal of Science, Section C, Volume 13 (1918), page 187.

It would seem that it might be worth while to examine the seeds of other Philippine species of *Shorea* and also of species of *Hopea*, as there are in the Philippines 21 species of *Shorea* and 13 of *Hopea*.

Family FLACOURTIACEAE

Genus PANGIUM

PANGIUM EDULE Reinw. PÁÑGI.

PITJOENG OIL

A description, figure, and the local names of this species are given in the bulletin on edible plants.

Pangium edule has seeds which yield about 50 per cent of pitjoeng, or samaun, oil having the following constants (Lewkowitsch) :

Specific gravity	0.937
Saponification value	178–183
Iodine value	89.94
Titer test of fatty acids	44.4

According to Lewkowitsch: *

The seeds contain a cyanogenetic glycoside of which some passes into the oil when it is prepared by the natives, and is only removed by prolonged boiling. The oil prepared in a very primitive fashion by the natives of Java, by heating the dry seeds and passing the mass between boards, is used as an edible oil.

Hefter † says that this oil is used as an illuminant and for making soap.

Family LECYTHIDACEAE

Genus BARRINGTONIA

BARRINGTONIA ASIATICA (L.) Kurz. BÓTONG.

Local names: *Balubitóon* (Guimaras Island); *bitóon* (Surigao); *booton*, *bótong* (Tayabas); *boton* (Tayabas, Camarines, Albay, Zamboanga); *lugo* (Cagayan); *palaupalau* (Negros).

BOTON OIL

Watt ‡ states that:

In the Moluccas a lamp-oil is said to be expressed from the seeds of this plant. (*Treasury of Botany.*)

---

* Lewkowitsch, J., Chemical technology and analysis of oils, fats, and waxes, Volume 2 (1914), page 496.

† Hefter, G., Technologie der Fette und Öle (1908), page 687.

‡ Watt, G., Dictionary of the economic products of India, Volume 1 (1885), page 403.

According to Hefter,* Schädler reports that the seeds of this species yield an oil which should be good for illumination. *Barringtonia asiatica* is a tree 8 to 15 meters in height. The leaves are 20 to 40 centimeters long, without individual stalks, shiny, larger near the apex than near the base, the apex rounded, and the base somewhat pointed. The flowers are very large. The petals are four in number, white, oblong, 7 to 8 centimeters long, and 3 to 4 centimeters wide. The stamens are very numerous, slender, united at the base, 10 to 12 centimeters long, white below, and shading to purple above. The fruit is sharply four- or rarely five-angled, 8 to 14 centimeters long, 8 to 12 centimeters thick, and contain a single large seed.

This species is distributed along the seashore throughout the Archipelago.

BARRINGTONIA RACEMOSA (L.) Blume.   PÚTAT.

Local names: *Kutkut timbalong* (Zamboanga); *paling* (Cagayan); *putad* (Mindoro); *pútat* (Bataan, Manila, Laguna, Tayabas, Camarines, Mindoro, Polillo, Ticao, Sibuyan, Negros, Cotabato, Zamboanga).

PÚTAT OIL

According to Hefter,* Schädler reports that the seeds of this species yield an oil which should be good for illumination.

Barringtonia racemosa is a shrub or small tree reaching a height of 10 meters. The leaves are crowded at the ends of the branches, smooth, 10 to 30 centimeters long, pointed at both ' ends; the margins toothed. The flowers are white, or pink. The petals are 2 to 2.5 centimeters long. The stamens are very numerous and are 3 to 4 centimeters long. The fruit is ovoid to oblong ovoid, 5 to 6 centimeters long, somewhat four-angled, and green or purple.

This species is found throughout the Philippines in open lowlands and thickets near the seashore.

Family COMBRETACEAE

Genus TERMINALIA

TERMINALIA CATAPPA L. (Fig. 55).   TALÍSAI.

Local names: *Almendra de Indias* (Spanish); *dalísai* (Cagayan); *logó* (Cagayan, Ilocos Norte and Sur, Abra, Union); *salaisáu* (Benguet); *salísai* (Zambales, Bataan); *savidug* (Batanes); *talísai* (Cagayan, Tarlac, Pampanga, Bulacan, Bataan, Rizal, Manila, Zambales, Laguna, Tayabas, Camarines, Mindoro, Albay, Sorsogon, Iloilo, Negros, Cotabato, Davao, Palawan); *talísi* (Basilan); *yalísai* (Tayabas).

---

* Hefter, G., Technologie der Fette und Öle, Volume 2 (1908), page 331.

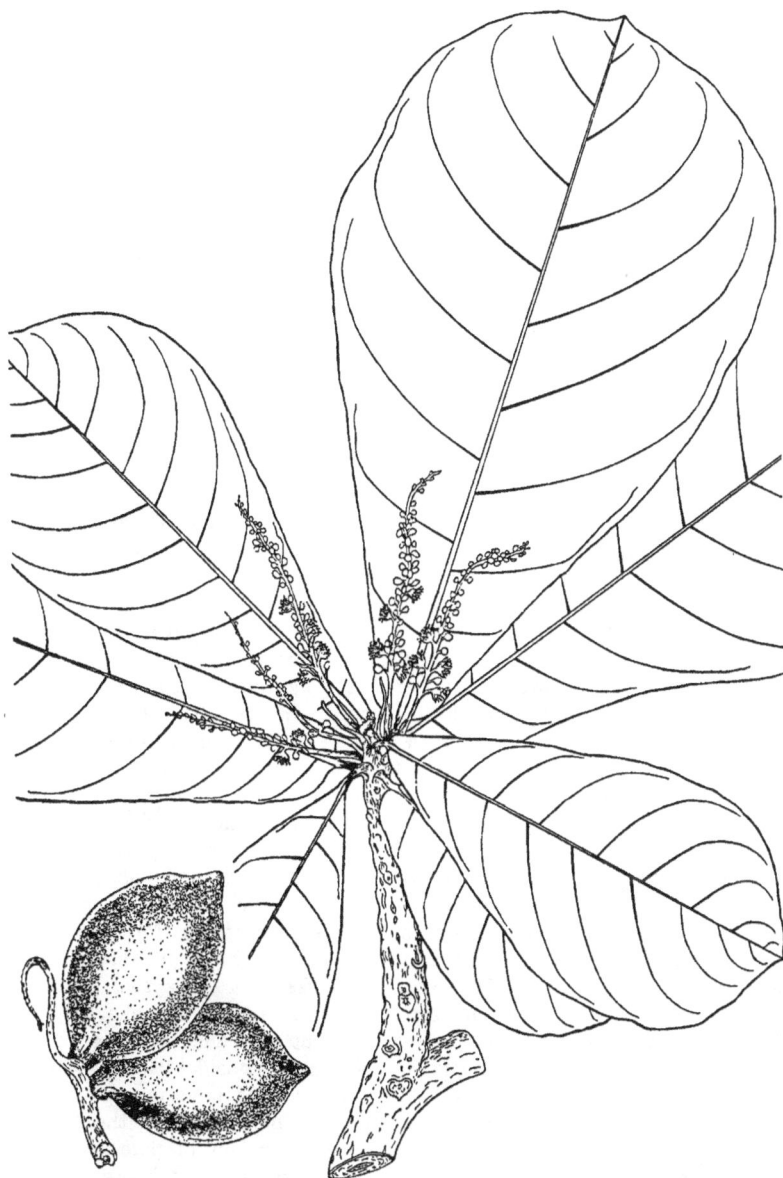

FIGURE 55. TERMINALIA CATAPPA (TALISAI), THE SOURCE OF INDIAN ALMOND OIL.
×½.

The kernel is edible and yields about 50 per cent of Indian almond oil, which is a sweet, savory, fixed oil. It closely resembles the oil of sweet almonds, for which it could well be substituted.

According to Lewkowitsch * the seeds of *Terminalia catappa* (country almond) contain 48.3 per cent of oil. Hooper † states that this oil has the following constants:

Specific gravity at 15° C.	0.9206
Melting point, °C.	3.5
Saponification value	203.04

	Per cent.
Iodine value	81.8
Insoluble acids+unsaponifiable	95.2
Titer test, °C.	42
Acid value	7.77

Concerning this oil, Watt ‡ say:

The kernels yield a valuable oil, similar to almond oil in flavour, odour, and specific gravity, but a little more deeply coloured; it deposits stearine on keeping. It possesses the advantage of not becoming rancid so readily as true almond oil, and if it could be produced cheaply would doubtless compete successfully with it. As the tree is abundant everywhere and the fruit could be doubtless obtained very cheaply, "Indian almond oil" appears to merit the attention of dealers. It was first brought prominently to notice by a Mr. A. T. Smith of Jessor, who in 1843 wrote to the Agr.-Horticultural Society of India an account of its properties and method of preparation. Oil, made experimentally by him, was expressed in the common native mill—a sort of pestle and mortar—from some fruit gathered during a few mornings from under the trees in the neighborhood. After a sufficient quantity had been gathered and allowed to dry in the sun for a few days, which facilitates breaking the nut, four coolies were set to work with small hammers, to separate the kernels from their shells. In four days they broke a sufficient quantity for one mill, *viz.*, 6 seers. This quantity put into the mill produced in three hours about 3 *pucka* seers of oil. Mr. Smith remarks that the actual pressing of the oil is of no consideration, since the value of the oil-cake, to feed pigs, etc., is sufficient to cover the expense, but that the breaking of the nuts is a tedious and costly operation, and is a consideration requiring particular attention, with a view to its reduction, if manufacture of the oil on an extensive scale should be attempted. The product of the experiment, filtered through blotting paper, was of the colour of pale sherry, a circumstance which Mr. Smith explains is due to the rind being allowed

* Lewkowitsch, J., Oils, fats, and waxes. Volume 3 (1915), page 451.

† Hooper, D., Annual report, Indian Museum, 1907–1908, page 13.

‡ Watt, G., A dictionary of the economic products of India, Volume 6, Part 4 (1893), page 23.

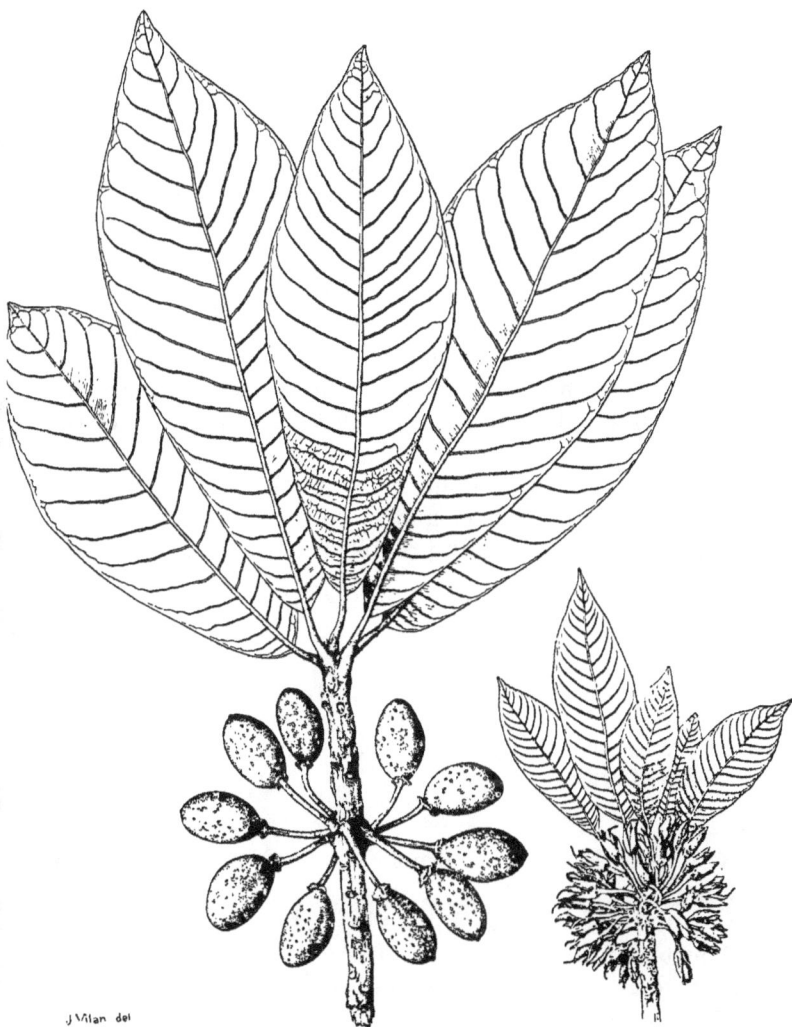

FIGURE 56. BASSIA BETIS (BÉTIS), THE SOURCE OF BÉTIS OIL.

to remain on the kernels. He concludes by remarking on the ornamental nature and utility of the tree for many other purposes, and recommends that it should be more extensively planted. A sample of the oil thus prepared was submitted for examination to Dr. Mouat, who reported as follows:—"I have compared the specimen with a good muster of the ordinary European almond oil in my possession, and find that in taste, smell, and specific gravity, the former is very similar to the latter, but is deeper in colour, becomes turbid in keeping, and deposits a quantity of white stearic matter. For most ordinary purposes, medicinal and otherwise, the former, I think, might profitably be substituted for the latter in this country, and, if expressed with greater care and freed from every impurity, might become an article of commercial value and importance" (*Journ. Agri.-Hort. Soc. Ind., ii.*). Though easily made edible and pleasant in flavour, it appears to have been entirely neglected by the Natives, who are ignorant as to its existence.

Terminalia catappa is a tree reaching a height of 25 meters. The leaves are 10 to 25 centimeters long, smooth, shiny, somewhat abruptly pointed at the tip, larger near the tip than near the base, tapering to a narrow, rounded or heart-shaped base. The flowers are small, white, and on axillary spikes 6 to 18 centimeters long.

This species is distributed near the seashore from northern Luzon to southern Mindanao, and is cultivated to some extent in and about Manila and many provincial towns as a shade tree.

Family SAPOTACEAE

Genus BASSIA

BASSIA BETIS (Blanco) Merr. (Figs. 56, 57). BÉTIS.

Local names: *Banitis* (Camarines); *bétis* (Rizal, Tayabas, Camarines); *betis-laláki* (Tayabas); *manílig* (Moro, Cotabato); *pásak* (Manila lumberyards); *piañga* (Cagayan, Isabela).

BÉTIS OIL

The fruit of this tree contains an oil used locally as an illuminant.

Bassia betis is a tree reaching a height of about 30 meters and a diameter of about 1 meter. The leaves are smooth on the upper surface and very hairy below. They are pointed at both ends and about 20 to 25 centimeters in length. The flowers and fruits are borne in rounded clusters. The stalks of the flowers and fruits are about 3 centimeters long. The flower, exclusive of the long style, is about 1.5 centimeters in length. The fruit is somewhat oval, and 3 or 4 centimeters in length.

This species is distributed from Luzon to Mindanao.

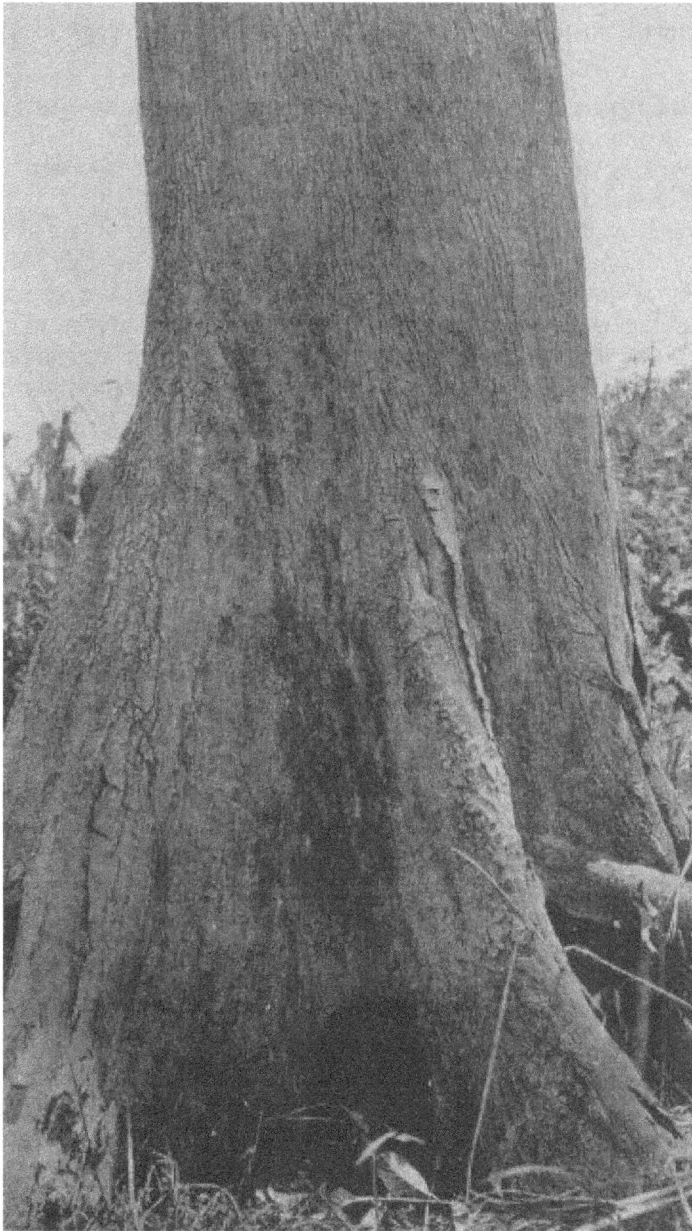

FIGURE 57. TRUNK OF BASSIA BETIS (BÉTIS).

Genus PALAQUIUM

PALAQUIUM PHILIPPENSE C. B. Rob.   MALAKMÁLAK.

MALAKMÁLAK OIL

A description, figure, and the local names of this species are given in the bulletin on edible plants.

According to Blanco * the seeds yield a limpid, odorous oil which is employed in food and as an illuminant.

Several writers mention an oil which is said to be obtained in other countries from *Palaquium oleosum* Blanco. What this plant may be is doubtful as Blanco described no such species and no such name is listed in Index Kewensis. The use of the name *Palaquium oleosum* may be due to confusion with *Palaquium oleiferum* Blanco, which is a synonym of *Palaquium philippense,* a species apparently confined to the Philippines.

Family APOCYNACEAE

Genus CERBERA

CERBERA MANGHAS Linn.   BARAIBÁI.

BARAIBÁI OIL

A description of this species and its local names are given in the bulletin on mangrove swamps.

Hefter † says that the seeds yield an illuminating oil.

Family PEDALIACEAE

Genus SESAMUM

SESAMUM ORIENTALE L. (Fig. 58).   SESAME or LIÑGÁ.

Local names: *Lañgis* (Pangasinan, Pampanga); *lañgá* (Camarines, Albay); *leñgñgá* or *liñgñgá* (Ilocos Norte and Sur, Abra, Pangasinan); *liñgá* (Tagalog provinces, Marinduque, Misamis, Cuyo Islands, Zamboanga); *luñgá* (Capiz and other Bisayan provinces).

BARAIBÁI OIL.

The whole seeds of *Sesamum orientale* are utilized locally by Chinese bakers in making various cakes and sweetmeats.

Sesame oil, also known as pil, or gingelly, is obtained by expressing the seeds of the sesame plant. The yield of oil thus obtained varies from about 50 to 57 per cent. The white or yellow seeded varieties furnish the best grade of oil, while the dark red, brown, or black seeded varieties give an oil of somewhat inferior grade. Sesame oil has a pale yellow color and a pleasant odor and taste.

---

* Blanco, M., Flora de Filipinas (1845), page 282.

† Hefter, G., Technologie der Fette und Öle, Volume 2, page 501.

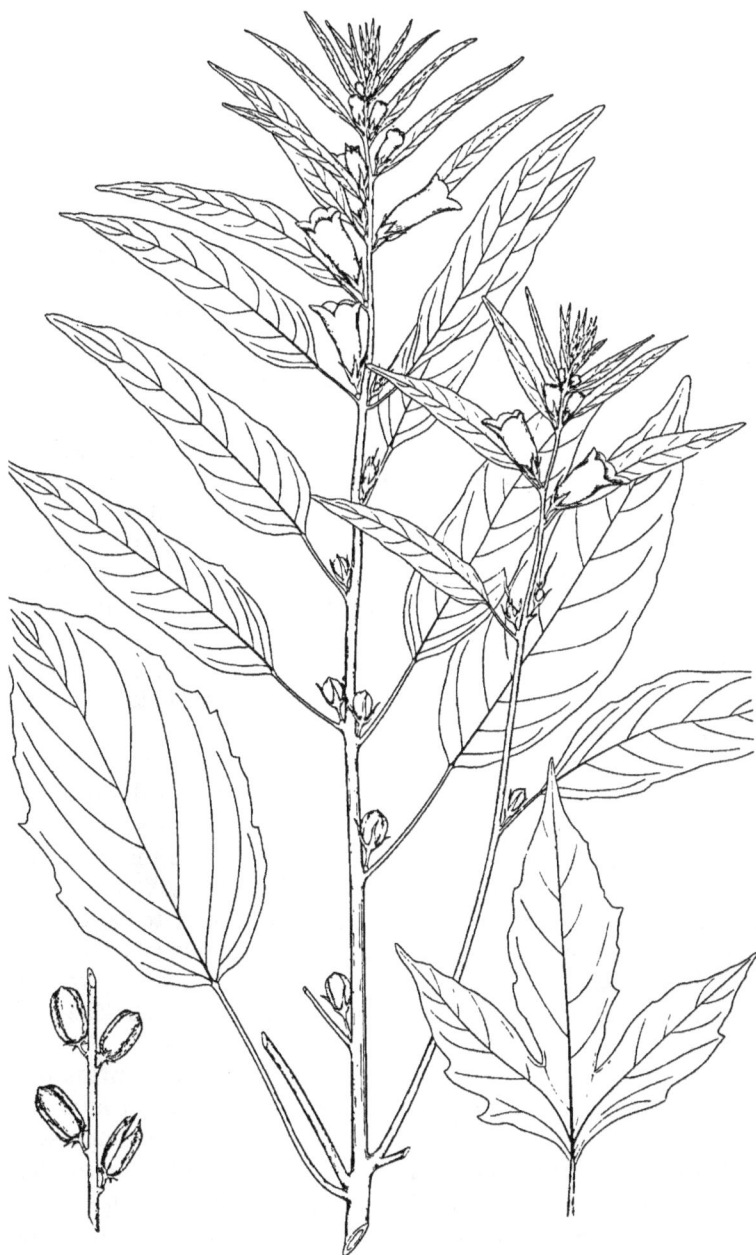

FIGURE 58. SESAMUM ORIENTALE, THE SOURCE OF SESAME OIL. ×½.

The Philippine exports of sesame seed and oil for several years
are given in Table 28.

TABLE 28.—*Amount and value of sesame seeds and oil exported from the
Philippines from 1914 to 1918.*

Year.	Seeds.		Oil.	
	Amount.	Value.	Amount.	Value.
	Kilo-grams.	*Pesos.*	*Kilo-grams.*	*Pesos.*
1914	53, 135	7, 328		
1915	62, 881	7, 464		
1916	316, 198	45, 675		
1917	168, 878	27, 558		
1918	120, 802	30, 661	6, 248	1, 250

The best quality of sesame oil is obtained from the first expression in the cold, and is used for edible purposes such as the
manufacture of margarine, which is an artificial butter or butter
substitute.   Oils of the second or third expression are employed
particularly in soap making.   After the free fatty acids have
been removed from the lower grades, they are likewise useful
for illuminating and lubricating purposes.

The oil cake contains about 9 per cent of oil.   It serves as an
excellent cattle food.   Oil cake which has been extracted with
solvents serves as fertilizer.

Before the war, sesame seeds were chiefly crushed on the con-
tinent of Europe.   In several continental countries the inclusion
of a certain quantity of sesame oil in margarine was compul-
sory, to facilitate its detection when used to adulterate butter.
This factor raised the price, with the result that the British
margarine producers substituted other oils, said to be cheaper
and equally good.   The seed is, however, now crushed in England, and it has been predicted that this practice will continue
and extend if the price of the seeds remains at about the same
level as that of the other oil seeds.*

In India and other eastern countries, the oil is expressed by
primitive methods and employed largely in cooking, for anointing
the body, and for lamps.   About 400,000 tons of sesame seeds
per year are used in India; in Burma about 100,000 tons.   The
average annual export from India is about 100,000 tons.   India
also exports about 180,000 tons of oil annually.   The total im-

---

* The oil-seed industry of Rhodesia. Bulletin of the Imperial Institute,
Volume 15 (1917), page 477.

ports of sesame into Europe in 1913 amounted to about 250,000 tons. In India the average value per ton of seeds is about 150 pesos. In Indo-China the yield of seeds varies from 300 to 800 kilos per hectare.*

According to The American Perfumer: †

The oil from the black variety of sesame is generally stated to be more suitable for medicinal purposes than the white. It is also extensively employed in the manufacture of Indian perfumes, and for this purpose the perfume is frequently extracted by the seeds direct—layers of the seeds being placed between layers of flowers, etc. Thus a favorite jasmine extract in India is made by layers of sesame seed wetted in water being placed alternately with layers of jasmine flowers, all being covered with a cloth and left for 12 to 18 hours, after which an oil is obtained that has all the scent of the flower.

As regards the composition of sesame oil, Mitchell ‡ says:

It consists, in the main, of the glycerides of oleic and linolic acid, with smaller quantities of the glycerides of solid fatty acids, including stearine, palmitin and myristin. The unsaponifiable matter (1 to 1.4 per cent.) consists of a phytosterol, a crystalline dextrorotatory substance, *sesamin*, and a substance termed *sesamol*, which reacts with furfural and hydrochloric acid.

Thorpe § in discussing the composition of sesame oil states:

Sesame oil contains from 12 to 14 p. c. of solid acids, the remainder consists of oleic and linoleic acids. Sesame oil is dextro-rotatory, a property which may supply a useful additional means of identifying the oil. The optical activity is no doubt due to the presence of phytosterol and sesamin which form the bulk of the unsaponifiable matter in sesame oil. In addition thereto, there occurs in the unsaponifiable matter a thick non-crystallisable oil which gives the characteristic colour reaction known as the "Baudouin."

Lewkowitsch ‖ gives the constants of sesame oil:

Specific gravity (15°), 0.9230 to 0.9237.
Solidifying point –4° to –6°.
Saponification value (Mgrms KOH) 188.5 to 190.4.
Iodine value 106.9 to 107.8.
Maumené test 63° to 72°.
Refractive index (15°), 1.4748–1.4762.
Oleo-refractometer (22°), +13° to +17°.
Butyro-refractometer (25°), 68° to 68.2°.

---

* Indian trade in oil seeds. Bulletin of the Imperial Institute, Volume 15 (1917), page 405.

† The American Perfumer, Volume 10 (1915–1916), page 244.

‡ Mitchell, C. A., Edible oils and fats (1918), page 69.

§ Thorpe, E., Dictionary of applied chemistry, Volume 4 (1912), page 661.

‖ Lewkowitsch, J., Oils, fats, and waxes, Volume 2 (1915), page 210.

Thorpe * states that sesame oil cake has the following average composition:

	Per cent.
Oil	14.63
Moisture	7.65
Proteins	36.14
Ash	13.17
Crude fiber	4.83
Carbohydrates	23.58

Sesamum orientale is an erect, annual herb 50 to 80 centimeters or more in height. The leaves are 3 to 10 centimeters long, the lower often lobed, the middle ones toothed, the uppermost almost entire. The petiole is from 1 to 5 centimeters long. The corolla is about 3 centimeters long, hairy, whitish, or with purplish, red, or yellow marks. The capsule is about 2.5 millimeters long and split half-way or quite to the base.

This plant is widely cultivated in the Philippines and is occasionally spontaneous. It is probably a native of tropical Africa, but is now widely distributed in tropical and subtropical countries.

The black-seeded variety of *Sesamum orientale* has been grown in the Philippine Islands as a minor crop for many years; the white-seeded variety, which produces a finer grade of oil, has been recently introduced.

---

* Thorpe, E., Dictionary of applied chemistry. Volume 4 (1912), page 661.

ESSENTIAL OILS

The natural essential oils are the volatile, odoriferous oils obtained from plants. By volatile is meant that if one of these oils is exposed to the air it will gradually evaporate. These volatile oils may occur in the bark, root, leaves, or other parts of the plant, but usually they are most abundant in the fruits or flowers. Many of these essential oils have a pleasant taste and a very fragrant odor, like that of fruits or flowers. They are employed extensively in the manufacture of various substances for which there is a great demand; as in perfumes, toilet waters, scents (face and sachet powders), and in essences which serve as flavoring materials for confectionery and for beverages like lemonade and liqueurs. They are also used in medicinal preparations to conceal nauseous odors and tastes.

Perfumes have been in vogue since the earliest times, and records show that the ancient Egyptians introduced perfumes in their religious services. In certain countries vast tracts of land are devoted to the cultivation of flowers from which fragrant perfumes are obtained. In southern France large quantities of various flowers are raised commercially for the production of natural perfumes. In the French Riviera district alone the annual revenue from cultivated flowers such as roses, carnations, and violets, is over ₱24,000,000. Roses are cultivated extensively in Bulgaria, while in the Philippines ilang-ilang is grown to a certain extent. In the Philippines there are a number of perfume plants which are the bases of considerable industries in other countries, but which are not so utilized in the Philippines. Among these are patchouli, lemon grass, and vetiver.

Various methods such as steam-distillation, extraction with fats (preparation of flower pomades), and extraction with volatile solvents are used to obtain the perfume oils from flowers.

As in the case of seed oils, the purity of essential oils is ascertained by determining certain essential-oil constants such as the specific gravity, optical rotation, and especially the ester number, as the value of many oils depends largely upon the presence of a quantity of certain esters. The real value of an oil, however, is determined by the exact odor it possesses. This

171

fragrance is due to certain chemical compounds, numbers of which exist in the flowers only in very minute quantities. Many of the chemical substances inherent in plants may be prepared synthetically. However, the odor of these synthetics is quite different from that of the flowers, for the latter's scent can be secured only when all the substances contained in the flower are combined in the proper proportions. The fragrant flower was the first perfume and still is the first. Although a large number of synthetic perfumes are manufactured, the consumption of natural perfumes is increasing. The former are frequently used to fortify the natural perfumes and are also mixed with them to produce new blends.

Family GRAMINEAE

Genus ANDROPOGON

ANDROPOGON CITRATUS DC.   TANGLÁD or LEMON GRASS.

Local names: *Barániw* (Pangasinan); *tañglád* (Tagalog, Bikol).

LEMON-GRASS OIL

This grass is frequently cultivated, especially in India and Ceylon, for its fragrant leaves. Bacon * remarks that in the Philippines:

It is cooked with stale fish to improve the taste and is used as a flavor in wines and various sauces and spices; it is also used medicinally, being applied to the forehead and face as a cure for headache, and an infusion is held in the mouth to alleviate the suffering of toothache.

The roots resemble ginger in flavor, though less pungent. They are used as a condiment and for perfuming hairwashes of gogo.

When the grass is distilled it yields commercial lemon-grass oil, or Indian verbena oil, which has a reddish-yellow color and the intense odor and taste of lemons. Lemon-grass oil is used in making perfumes, especially ionone (synthetic essence of violets).

According to Hood † about 100,000 pounds of lemon-grass oil are used annually in the United States and the consumption of it for the manufacture of ionone and other perfumery purposes is continually increasing. He describes the distillation of the grass as follows:

---

* Bacon, R. F., Philippine terpenes and essential oils, III. Philippine Journal of Science, Section A, Volume 4 (1909), page 111.

† Hood, S. C., Possibility of the commercial production of lemon-grass oil in the United States. United States Department of Agriculture Bulletin No. 442 (1917).

The apparatus required for the distillation of lemon-grass oil does not differ from that in general use for the distillation of other volatile oils. Before distilling the plants it has been found advisable to run them through a fodder cutter, in order to permit closer packing in the retort. From the data at hand it is estimated that if the plants are cut into 2-inch lengths a retort will hold 100 pounds of material for every 6 cubic feet of space, but if the plants are put in whole the quantity which the retort can hold will be somewhat less. The closer packing, however, in no way facilitates distillation.

In a retort having a capacity of 30 cubic feet a charge of 3,000 pounds can be distilled in 2 to 2½ hours by the steam which may be readily generated in a small farm boiler, and by the use of a larger volume of steam the time can be much reduced.

After the oil has been distilled it should be freed from water so far as possible in a separatory funnel, then dried by shaking with anhydrous calcium chloride, and filtered. It should be stored in well-filled air-tight containers in as cold a place as possible until ready to be shipped to market. The shipping can be done in new and clean tin cans without injury to the product.

Leach,* in discussing lemon extracts, states:

The flavor of the cheap extracts is sometimes reinforced by the addition of such substances as citral, oil of citronella, and oil of lemon grass, but minute quantities only of these pungent materials can be used, not exceeding 0.33 per cent in the case of citral, and 0.1 per cent in the case of the two last mentioned oils.

According to Askinson,† essence of lemon grass consists of 2 ounces of lemon-grass oil dissolved in 1 gallon of alcohol.

Lemon-grass oil consists largely of citral and contains also small quantities of various substances such as methyl heptenone, and the terpenes, limonene and dipentene. The exact value of the oil depends chiefly upon the amount of citral it contains. High-grade oils contain about 70 to 80 per cent of citral. This is an aldehyde which occurs not only in lemon-grass oil, but also in lemon oil (the oil obtained from lemon peel) and in many other natural essential oils.

Bacon investigated lemon grass grown at the Government experimental station at Lamao, Bataan, in unfertilized soil. Concerning his results on these plots of grass he states:

Lamao.—Planted February 14, 1908. First cutting July 29, 1908. Obtained 432 kilos grass, from 57 square meters of ground, distilled two days after cutting, the yield was 900 grams of oil (0.2 per cent) of the following properties: Specific gravity, $\frac{30°}{4°} = 0.894$; $N \frac{30°}{D} = 1.4857$; $A \frac{30°}{D} = +8.1$; citral = 79 per cent; Schimmel's test passes the oil.

---

* Leach, A. E. Food inspection and analysis (1914), page 872.

† Askinson, G. W., Perfumes and cosmetics, page 161.

Bacon thought that lemon grass should be considered as a ' possible catch crop for the first few years of new Philippine plantations. He did not recommend it as a permanent crop on account of the limited demand for the oil. The grass from which oil has been extracted is burned under the distilling boiler and the ashes distributed over the fields as fertilizers. The exhausted grass is also used for making paper.

Lemon grass is a tufted perennial with leaves up to 1 meter in length and 1.4 centimeters in width. It is widely distributed, but not extensively cultivated in the Philippines and does not grow outside of cultivation.

ANDROPOGON NARDUS var. HAMATULUS Hack.

CITRONELLA OIL

The typical form of this species is cultivated in India, Ceylon, and other tropical countries for the essential oil obtained from it. It probably could be cultivated in the Philippines also. When this grass is distilled it yields a pale yellow oil, which has a very strong odor and is known commercially as citronella oil.

As the variety *hamatulus*, which occurs in the Philippines, has not been investigated chemically, it is not certain that it will yield citronella oil.

On account of its low price, citronella oil is used chieflly for perfuming cheap soaps and also as a protection against the bites of insects. An ointment containing 25 per cent of oil of citronella is an excellent protection against mosquitoes. · According to Parry * pure citronella oil has the following constants:

Specific gravity	0.900 to 0.915
Rotation	0° to –15°
Sp. gr. of 1st 10 per cent (distilled at 20–40 mm.)	above 0.858
Refractive index of same at 20°	above 1.4570
Solubility in 80 per cent alcohol	to pass Schimmel's test
Geraniol and citronella	above 58 per cent
(Calculated as total geraniol).	

Parry describes methods for preparing pure citronella oil. He also discusses methods for determining the purity and the presence of adulterants.

Askinson † states that essence of citronella contains three ounces of citronella oil dissolved in one gallon of alcohol.

---

* Parry, E. J. Chemistry of essential oils and artificial perfumes, (1908), page 171.

† Askinson, G. W., Perfumes and cosmetics (1915), page 161.

, The variety *hamatulus* is of very local occurrence in the Philippines, is nowhere cultivated, and is apparently not used in the Archipelago. It is distributed from the northern to the southern limits of the Philippines.

ANDROPOGON ZIZANIOIDES (L.) Urb. (Fig. 59). VETIVER or MORAS.

Local names: *Amóra* (Cebu); *amóras* (Ilocos Norte); *aniás* or *aniás de móras* (Pampanga); *anís de móro* (Ilocos Sur, Abra); *gerón, girón* (Iloilo); *ilíb* (Pampanga); *móra* or *móras* (Pampanga, Tarlac, Rizal, Manila, Laguna, Camarines, Albay, Sorsogon, Antique, Cebu, Occidental Negros); *rimódas* (Capiz); *rimóra* (Zambales); *rimóras* (Camarines); *tres móras* (Capiz).

VETIVER OIL

Oil obtained from the roots of this grass is known as *vetiver* and also as *cuscus*. The oil is obtained by steam-distilling the roots which are first macerated in water. It has been employed as an aromatic, carminative and diaphoretic. It is used considerably as a constituent of high grade perfumes and also as a perfume fixative, which makes the odors less volatile and more lasting.

According to Askinson,* the roots are used in India for making fragrant mats, while shavings are employed for filling sachet bags. The odor of the roots is somewhat similar to that of sandal wood. Fans made of the roots are sold in oriental-curio shops in the United States under the name of "sandal-root" fans. Piesse † states that in Calcutta, vetiver (vitivert or kus-kus) is made into awnings and sunshades. During the hot season the shades are sprinkled with water, the evaporation of which cools the apartment, while the atmosphere is perfumed with the fragrant odor.

In the Philippines, the roots are woven into fans which are prized on account of their agreeable odor. The stalks are also used for making hats, while the leaves are sometimes employed for thatching.

According to Watt,‡ the roots of *Andropogon zizanioides*—

* * * When distilled with water yield a fragrant Oil (known in European trade as *Vetiver*, which is used as a perfume and for flavouring sherbet. It commands a high price in Europe, being employed in many favourite scents. It is the most viscid of essential oils, and hence its sparing volatility .is taken advantage of in fixing other perfumes. The oil is hardly, if ever, exported from India, European supplies being either locally

---

* Askinson, G. W., Perfumes and cosmetics (1915), pages 54, 173, 225.

† Piesse, C. H., Art of perfumery (1891), page 233.

‡ Watt, George, The commercial products of India (1908), page 1106.

made from the Indian roots or derived from Réunion. According to Piesse,⁴ the yield is about 10 oz. per cwt.; other observers have found it to vary from 0.2 to 3.5 per cent. * * *

The odor of vetiver, Parry * says, does not resemble that of orris root, but has a similar effect in perfumery. Vetiver essence is obtained by treating three pounds of the dried roots with one gallon of alcohol. It is used in making various high-grade bouquet perfumes. Parry states that from the standpoint of practical perfumery vetiver oil is said to blend excellently with the odors of orris root and cassie flowers. Askinson says that vetiver essence consists of 2 ounces of vetiver oil dissolved in one gallon of alcohol, and vetiver sachet powder of 2 pounds of vetiver roots, 15 grains of musk, and 20 grains of civet.

According to Bacon,† the distillation of the greater part of vetiver oil is carried on in Europe. Neither the roots nor the oil appear to be exported from the Philippines. The roots are sold in the large public markets of the Philippines in small lots at from 15 to 25 centavos per kilo. They are usually laid away with clothing to impart a pleasant odor. Bacon believed that the cultivation and distillation of this grass offered commercial possibilities in the Philippines.

Parry ‡ states that Schimmel investigated this oil and obtained the following results:

Specific gravity	1.019 to 1.027
Optical rotation	+25° to +26°
Ester number (as per cent KOH)	7 to 8
Solubility in 80 per cent alcohol	1 in 1½ to 2

Singh § distilled seven samples of vetiver roots and found that the yield of oil obtained varied from 0.45 to 1.14 per cent The resin contained in the oil was eliminated by redistillation and the refined oil then gave a negative optical rotation (–30.65°).

An extensive investigation of vetiver oil and a review of the literature on this subject has been made by Semmler, Risse, and Schröter.‖ The oil used by these investigators was prepared by Schimmel. They obtained from vetiver oil various substances

---

* Parry, E. J., Chemistry of essential oils and artificial perfumes (1908), page 186.

† Bacon, R. F., Philippine terpenes and essential oils, III. Philippine Journal of Science, Section A, Volume 4 (1909), page 118.

‡ Parry, E. J., Chemistry of essential oils and artificial perfumes (1908), page 186.

§ Singh, Puran, American Perfumer, Volume 10 (1915–1916), page 133.

‖ Semmler, F. W., Risse, F., and Schröter, F., Berichte der Deutschen Chemischen Gesellschaft. Volume 45, II (1912), page 153.

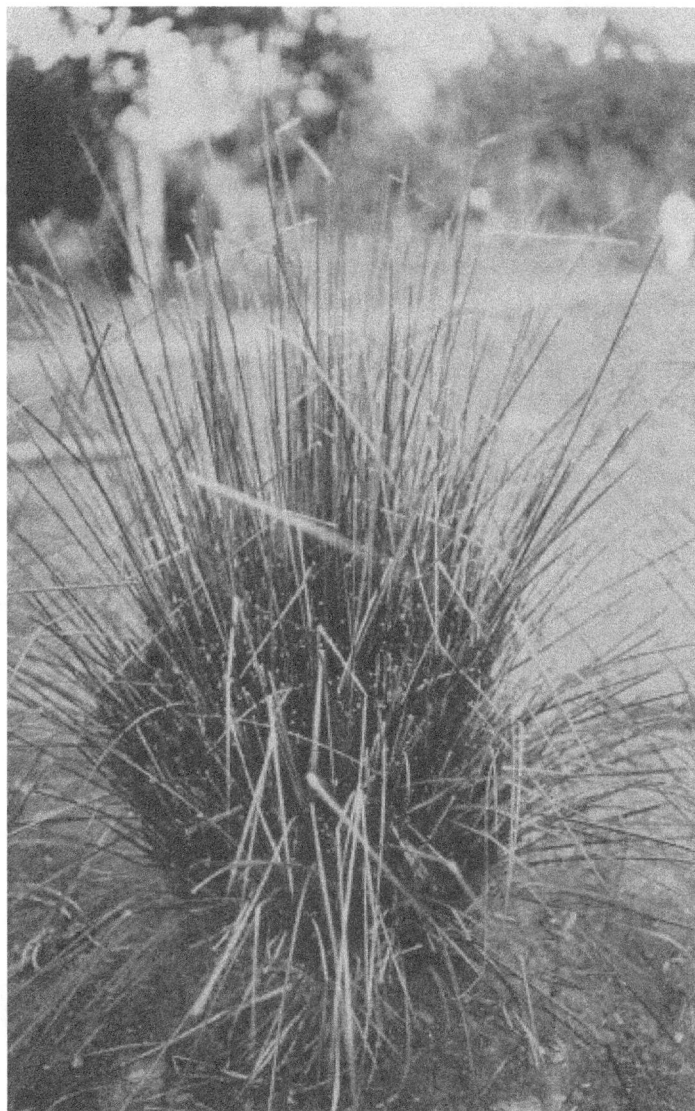

FIGURE 59. ANDROPOGON ZIZANIOIDES (VETIVER OR MORAS), THE SOURCE OF VETIVER OIL.

168837——12

such as the vetivenes, vetivenol, vetivenic acid, vetivenyl ace‑tate, and similar compounds.

Bacon * reports the results of his investigation on vetiver as follows:

(1) Thirty kilos of fresh vetiver roots were distilled for two working days (seven hours each) with steam, the condensed water being continually poured back over the roots, and the oil collected in a little petroleum ether to effect easier separation from the water, as the vetiver oil has almost the same specific gravity as water. The petroleum ether was distilled *in vacuo* and there were thus separated 327 grams of a light yellow oil (1.09 per cent) which had a very strong, pleasant odor and the following properties: Specific gravity, $\frac{30}{4}$ $=0.9935$; A $\frac{30^\circ}{D}$ $=+32.1$; N $\frac{30^\circ}{D}=1.5212$ saponification number $=47.4$

The roots used in the above experiment were obtained from small gardens about Manila and were crushed between the rollers of a sugar mill before being distilled. Such a crushing of the roots seems to improve the yield of oil.

(2) Thirty-one kilos of fresh roots, uncrushed, on distillation as above gave 140 grams oil (0.3 per cent).

(3) Six kilos of dried roots, uncrushed, gave by extraction with ligroin 14 grams of an oil which had only a very slight vetiver odor.

(4) Eighty-one kilos of dry *moras* which had been stored in jute sacks for about three months after harvesting, were distilled with steam with continuous cohobation and yielded 370 grams of oil (0.456 per cent) of an intense odor and brown color. This oil had the following properties: Specific gravity, $\frac{30}{4^\circ}$ $=0.9964$; N $\frac{30^\circ}{D}=1.5163$; A $\frac{30^\circ}{D}=+32.1$; saponification number $=60.0$.

It is to be noted that this oil with a higher saponification number has a much stronger odor than that obtained in experiment 1 given above (saponification number $=47.4$

(5) A plot of well-fertilized ground containing 150 square meters was planted with vetiver grass. In six months time the plants had flowered and reached maturity; they were then removed, giving 270 kilos of roots, or at the rate of over 18,000 kilos per crop per hectare. However, it was found when these roots were transferred to the laboratory, that they had lost most of their odor, and they gave so small a yield of oil as not to make it worth while to distill them. Some of these plants had been pulled up from time to time and tested for their oil content; they seem to contain the oil up to the time of flowering.

These preliminary experiments seemed to indicate that the proper time for harvesting is about three months after planting, at which time, of course, the yield of roots is not nearly so heavy. The oil in the roots is a protection, and is withdrawn when the plant flowers and seeds. We have planted all of our vetiver by simply burying pieces of divided root tufts in the ground. We have as yet made no experiments on the propagation of the grass from the seed. It was found that the roots can very con-

---

* Bacon, R. F., Philippine terpenes and essential oils, III. Philippine Journal of Science, Section A, Volume 4 (1909), page 119.

veniently be harvested by washing away the soil with a stream of water, catching detached rootlets with a coarse screen. One hundred plants of the above lot, treated in this manner, gave 60 kilos of roots (wet), and 100 plants at Parañaque in a sandy beach soil, gave 23 kilos of roots. The latter were presumably three to four months old and contained a large percentage of oil.

Andropogon zizanioides is a coarse, erect, tufted, perennial grass 1 to 2 meters in height. It has fragrant, fibrous roots. The leaves, arranged in two rows, are about 1 meter long, 1 centimeter or less in width, and folded. The panicles are terminal, erect or greenish, and about 20 centimeters long.

This grass abounds in all parts of the Archipelago. It is identical with the *khus-khus* or *khas-khas* of India. It grows abundantly in Burma and is also found in Réunion, Mauritius, and the West Indies.

Family ARACEAE

Genus ACORUS

ACORUS CALAMUS L. LUBIGÁN or SWEET FLAG.

Local names: *Acóro* (Spanish); *bueng* (Pampango); *lubigán* (Tagalog, Bíkol, Bisaya); *dálau* (Ilocos Sur, Abra, Union); *dárau, dengau* (Bontoc).

CALAMUS OIL

The rhizome of sweet flag has an agreeable, aromatic odor, and when powdered is used for sachet and toilet powders. The rhizome yields calamus oil when distilled. This oil is used for the preparation of aromatic cordials and liqueurs, for flavoring beer, and also in making perfumes. Throughout the Malayan region and the Philippines it is highly prized for medicinal purposes.

Askinson * gives the essence of calamus as consisting of 1¾ ounces of calamus oil dissolved in 5 quarts of alcohol. Although this essence has a pleasant odor, it is not a very valuable perfume and is usually employed as a basis for cheap perfumery preparations.

Parry † states that Schimmel obtained 0.8 per cent of oil from the dried rhizome, while the fresh rhizome yielded about 2.0 per cent. According to Parry, a thorough chemical investigation of this oil has not been made. However, it is supposed to contain pinene and a sesquiterpene. Schimmel found that the specific gravity varied from 0.960 to 0.970 and the optical rotation from + 10° to + 35°. Oil from the Japan calamus root, however, gave a specific gravity of 1.000. Pure samples of calamus

---

* Askinson, G. W., Perfumes and cosmetics, (1915).

† Parry, E. J., The chemistry of essential oils and artificial perfumes. (1908).

oil are soluble in 90 per cent alcohol and should yield no distillate below 170°.

Acorus calamus has stout, branched, aromatic rhizomes. The leaves are flat, smooth, 25 to 60 centimeters long, and 1 to 1.5 centimeters wide. The spathe is green, much elongated, and similar in shape to the leaves. The spadix is 3 to 5 centimeters long, 1 centimeter or less in diameter, and bears many flowers. This species occurs throughout the Philippines as a cultivated plant. In the Mountain Province, Luzon, at and above an altitude of 1,400 meters, it is sometimes found growing wild in swamps in great abundance. However, this plant has apparently been introduced into the Philippines.

Family ZINGIBERACEAE

Genus CURCUMA

CURCUMA LONGA L.   DILÁU OR TURMERIC.

Local names: *Áñge* (Pampanga); *azafrán* (Spanish in Zamboanga); *barák* (Cuyo Islands); *dálau* (Iloko in Cagayan); *diláu* (Bataan, Rizal, Manila, Laguna, Batangas, Tayabas); *dilau-pulá* (Laguna); *duláu* (Leyte, Capiz, Iloilo, Cuyo Islands); *kalauág* (Camarines, Albay, Zambales); *kulálau* (Pangasinan); *kúnig* (Ilocos Sur, Cagayan); *luyang-diláu* (Batangas).

DILÁU OIL

The rhizomes of *Curcuma longa* are used extensively in the Philippines as a condiment and for food coloration and also as an ingredient of curry.

Bacon * found that when 123 kilos of roots were distilled, 290 grams of a brown-colored oil were obtained. The constants of this oil were as follows: Specific gravity, $\frac{30°}{30°}$ =0.930; refractive index N $\frac{30°}{D}$ =1.5030; optical rotation, A $\frac{30°}{D}$ =8°.6; ester number, 81; miscible with 75 per cent alcohol.

Turmeric (curcumin) is the yellow coloring matter (dye) obtained from the rhizomes of *Curcuma longa*.

It is not exported from the Philippines at the present time. The value of the importations into the United States in 1907 was 26,252 dollars, the greater part being from Burma.

Curcuma longa resembles *Curcuma zedoaria*, but its flowering shoot is borne within the tuft of leaves and not directly from the rootstock as is that of *Curcuma zedoaria*. It has 5 or 6 thin, smooth, pale-green, pointed leaves, which are about 45 centi-

---

* Bacon, R. F., Philippine terpenes and essential oils, IV. Philippine Journal of Science, Section A, Volume 5 (1910), page 262.

meters long and 12 to 18 centimeters wide. The flowering spike is 12 to 20 centimeters long and borne on a stalk of about the same length. The bracts are 2 to 3 centimeters long, spreading, recurved, pale green, the terminal one sometimes rosy.

This species is distributed from northern Luzon to Mindanao, and is locally abundant in the settled areas. *Curcuma longa* is commonly cultivated and the wild plants are probably descendants of planted ones.

CURCUMA ZEDOARIA Bosc.   BARÁK or ZEDOARY.

Local names: *Alimpuying* (Negros Oriental); *barák* (Bataan, Mindoro); *ganda* (Zambales); *koniko* (Bontoc); *luyaluyáhan, tamo* (Rizal); *lampoyáng* (Guimaras Island); *tamahílan* (Camarines).

ZEDOARY OIL

The stout, fleshy, aromatic rootstocks when dry are called zedoary. The roots yield a volatile oil when distilled with water, and contain a pungent, soft resin and bitter extractive. They have an odor somewhat like that of ginger.

Watt * says that the rhizomes constitute one of the most important articles of native perfumery in India. The root is also used medicinally. According to the nineteenth edition of the United States Dispensatory, zedoary is a warm, stimulating aromatic, serviceable in flatulent colic and debility of the digestive organs, but is now little used, as it produces no effect which cannot be as well or better obtained from ginger.

Bacon † found that 160 kilograms of rhizomes when chopped and steam-distilled gave 400 grams (0.25 per cent) of a light yellow oil which had the following properties:—Specific gravity, $\frac{30°}{4°} = 0.993$; refractive index, $N\frac{30°}{D} = 1.5070$; optical rotation, $A\frac{30°}{D} = 1°.10$; saponification number, 2; soluble in two or more volumes of 80 per cent alcohol. This oil was distilled *in vacuo* (7 millimeters) and the distillate separated into fractions. Fraction 4, (140° to 160°) and fraction 5, (160° to 166°), gave 131 grams of oil which solidified to a beautiful white, crystalline compound, which Bacon thought was probably a sesquiterpene alcohol.

Curcuma zedoaria is an erect herb with a stout, fleshy, aromatic rootstock. The leaves usually grow in pairs and are green, often with a purplish blotch in the center. They are from 25 to 70

---

* Watt, The commercial products of India, 1908.

† Bacon, R. F., Philippine terpenes and essential oils, IV. Philippine Journal of Science, Section A, Volume 5 (1910), page 261.

centimeters long and 8 to 15 centimeters wide. The flower stalks spring directly from the rootstocks and not from the leaf tuft, and often appear before the leaves. The spike is cylindrical, 5 to 8 centimeters in diameter and 10 to 15 centimeters long, and is composed of numerous somewhat spreading, rounded bracts, the lower of which are green and more or less tipped with pink, the upper ones usually longer and purple, each containing several flowers, of which the lower open first. The corolla tube is about 2 centimeters long, yellowish-white, sometimes tinged with purple.

This species is probably a native of India, but is now widely distributed in the warmer parts of the eastern hemisphere. It is common and widely distributed in thickets and open places in the settled parts of the Philippines.

Genus ZINGIBER

ZINGIBER OFFICINALE Bosc.   GINGER.

Local names: *Agát* (Pangasinan); *gengibre* (Spanish); *láya* (Pampanga); *layá* (Abra, Ilocos Norte and Sur, Capiz, Iloilo); *la-yá* or *lay-á* (Zambales, Camarines, Albay, Sorsogon); *lúya* (Tarlac, Bulacan, Bataan, Rizal, Laguna, Manila, Batangas, Tayabas, Mindoro, Marinduque); *luy-á* (Albay, Iloilo, Occidental Negros, Misamis, Cuyo Islands).

GINGER

Zingiber officinale is cultivated in all parts of the Philippines, but never on a large scale, and is not exported. The dried root of this plant has a pungent, aromatic odor and is commonly known as ginger. Ginger is used as a condiment and as a flavoring agent. It is also employed medicinally as an aromatic stimulant and carminative, and is given in cases of dyspepsia and flatulent colic. It is utilized in the manufacture of ginger beer and ginger ale and also as a spice and a confection.

Ginger consists essentially of a volatile oil, a resin, and starch. Its pungency is due to the resin it contains, while the aroma is given by the volatile oil. An analysis of Calcutta ginger quoted by Leach * gave the following results:

Water	9.60
Ash	7.02
Volatile oil	2.27
Fixed oil and resin	4.58
Starch	49.34
Crude fibre	7.45
Albuminoids	6.30
Undetermined	13.44
Nitrogen	1.01

- * Leach, A. E., Food inspection and analysis (1914), page 446.

Oil of ginger is obtained by distilling the ginger root. It has a greenish-yellow color and is very aromatic though not pungent. It is slightly soluble in alcohol. Ginger oil, and also the alcoholic extract of ginger roots, are used for flavoring beverages. Bacon * distilled two lots of Philippine ginger roots and examined the distillates. He describes his results as follows:

* * * I made two experiments on the distillation of native ginger roots. In the first one, 50 kilos of the chopped roots gave only 25 grams of oil. For the second, 132 kilos were purchased in the market at Malabon at 22 centavos, (11 cents United States currency) per kilo and immediately distilled. There were obtained 95 grams (0.072 per cent) of a light yellow oil, having the odor of ginger and also a strong smell, much like that of orange-peel oil.

This oil had the following properties:

Specific gravity $\frac{30°}{30°} = 0.8850$.

Refractive index, $N_D^{30°} = 1.4830$.

Optical rotation, $A_D^{30°} = -5.°9.†$

Saponification number, 14.

It is easily and completely soluble in two or more volumes of 90 per cent alcohol.

It is seen that oil from the Philippine ginger differs quite markedly in its properties from that distilled from the Jamaica or African varieties and resembles some Japanese oils examined by Schimmel and Company in its ready solubility in 90 per cent alcohol, and its negative optical rotation.

Family MAGNOLIACEAE

Genus MICHELIA

MICHELIA CHAMPACA L. (Fig. 60). CHAMPÁKA.

Local names: *Champákang-pulá* (Manila); *sampáka* (Rizal).

CHAMPÁKA OIL

Oil obtained from the flowers of this species is used as a perfume.

Roure-Bertrand Fils ‡ state in their bulletin that the perfume of Philippine champaka flowers is stronger and sweeter than that of the flowers obtained from Singapore, Penang or Colombo.

---

* Bacon, R. F., Philippine terpenes and essential oils, IV. Philippine Journal of Science, Section A, Volume 5 (1910), page 259.

† In the original, the minus sign is omitted, apparently through error, since Bacon says, in the body of the paper, that the oil has a negative rotation.

‡ Bulletin of Roure-Bertrand Fils, Volume 1 (1909), page 26.

In experimenting with champaka flowers it is necessary to work rapidly because a few hours after picking, the flowers turn brown and begin to lose their fragrance. The oil obtained from these flowers has been investigated by Bacon * and by Brooks.† According to Bacon:

The yield appears to be over 0.2 per cent. The crude oil on standing separated a large amount of a crystalline solid. This was filtered and an additional quantity of it was again separated by the addition of ether, in which the solid is quite insoluble. The remaining oil, after standing for some weeks in the laboratory, continued to solidify until it gradually became semisolid. The second solid which separated was amorphous and appeared to be resinous in nature. If this semisolid extract is treated with 70 per cent alcohol, about half of it separates in the form of the amorphous, brown, odorless body. This was filtered and the filtrate concentrated at 40° *in vacuo* until a brown oil separated, which had a very fine odor of champaca, and was readily soluble in 70 per cent alcohol or stronger. Our oil had the following constants: Specific gravity, $\frac{30°}{30°}$, 0.9543; refractive index, $N\frac{30°}{D}$, 1.4550; saponification number, 160. Another oil had specific gravity, $\frac{30°}{30°}$, 1.020; refractive index, $N\frac{30}{D}$, 1.4830; saponification number, 180. The second oil had the finer odor. The oils were too dark to permit of determinations of the optical activity. * * *

Fifty grams of champaka oil (soluble in 70 per cent alcohol, ester number 180) were saponified with 10 grams potassium hydrate in 100 cubic centimeters of 95 per cent alcohol. After heating for one hour with a reflux condenser, two volumes of water were added; 4.5 grams of an amorphous solid separated. This was filtered and the filtrate was separated into neutral, acid, and phenol fractions. By saponification the champaka oil loses all of its characteristic odor, which therefore must be due to esters.

The phenol fraction (1.5 grams) proved to consist principally of iso-eugenol, as benzoyl iso-eugenol melting at 103° could be obtained from it. The total acid fraction weighed 15 grams. None of this acid boils below 140° at 40 millimeters; hence there is no methyl ethyl acetic acid. No acids have as yet been identified.

The neutral portion weighed 23 grams and had an odor somewhat similar to that of oil of bay.

Bacon found that the solid which crystallizes from the freshly prepared oil, after repeated crystallization from benzene and petroleum ether, forms odorless, white crystals.

Brooks examined two samples of champaka oil and obtained the constants recorded in Table 29.

---

* Bacon, R. F., Philippine terpenes and essential oils, III, Philippine Journal of Science, Section A, Volume 4 (1909), page 131; IV, Volume 5 (1910), page 262.

† Brooks, B. T., New Philippine essential oils. Philippine Journal of Science, Section A, Volume 6 (1911), page 333.

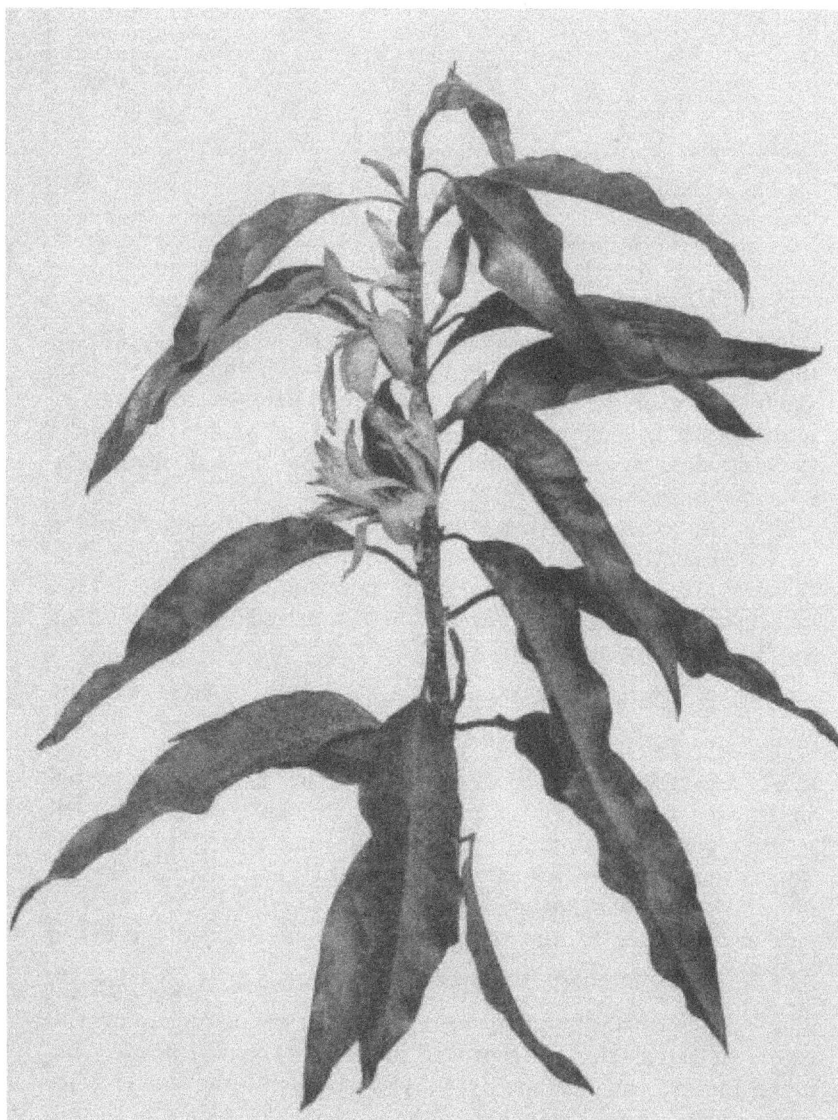

FIGURE 60. MICHELIA CHAMPACA (CHAMPÁKA), THE SOURCE OF CHAMPÁCA OIL.

TABLE 29.—*Constants of champaka oil.*

Constants.	Specimen No.	
	I.	II.
Specific gravity $\frac{30°}{30°}$	0.904	0.9107
Refractive index $N\frac{30°}{D}$	1.4640	1.4688
Ester number	124	146
Ester number after acetylating		199

According to Brooks, when champaka oil is heated, a large part of it is polymerized to resin. The oil obtained by steam-distilling consists largely of cineol. The solid which crystallizes from the freshly prepared oil is probably a ketone compound. In addition to iso-eugenol, the essential oil of yellow champaka flowers contains benzoic acid, benzyl alcohol, benzaldehyde, cineol, and p-cresol methyl ether.

Michelia champaca is a small tree with spear-shaped leaves, 12 to 20 centimeters long and 2.5 to 6 centimeters wide. The flowers are yellowish brown, very fragrant, and from 4 to 5 centimeters in length. They are highly prized by the Filipinos and by them are made into necklaces.

MICHELIA LONGIFLORA Blume.   CHAMPÁKANG-PUTÍ.

CHAMPÁKANG-PUTÍ OIL

Champaka oil obtained from this species has been exported to Europe from Java. According to Brooks * the purified oil is dark green in color. It possesses an intensely sweet, almost nauseating odor, which is very different from that of the oil obtained from the flowers of *Michelia champaca*.

The constants of the oil are as follows: Specific gravity, 0.897; ester number, 180.0; refractive index, $N\frac{30}{D} = 1.4470$. The above constants point to a rather large per cent of the esters of fatty acids. According to Brooks the oil contains linaloöl, methyl eugenol, methyl-ethyl-acetic acid, and acetic acid. The odor of the oil is chiefly that of the methyl or ethyl ester of methyl-ethyl-acetic acid.

Michelia longiflora is a small tree with white flowers. It is a native of Java and is occasionally cultivated in Manila.

---

* Brooks, B. T., New Philippine essential oils. Philippine Journal of Science, Volume 6 (1911), page 333.

Family ANNONACEAE

Genus CANANGIUM

CANANGIUM ODORATUM (Lam.) Baill. (Figs. 61–62). ILANG-ÍLANG.
Local names: *Alañgígan* (Ilocos Norte and Sur, Abra, Lepanto); *ala-ñgílan* (Mindoro); *anañgílan* (Surigao); *anañgíran* (Manobo); *búrak* (Leyte); *ilang-ílang* (Ilocos Sur, Zambales, Tayabas, Bataan, Rizal, Manila, Laguna, Mindoro, Balabac Island, Masbate, Guimaras Island, Ticao Island, Davao, Surigao); *tañgíd, tañgít* (Camarines, Albay, Sorsogon).

ILANG-ÍLANG OIL

Ilang-ilang * oil is obtained by steam-distilling the flowers of *Canangium odoratum*, in perfume literature sometimes called "the flower of flowers." The best grade of distilled oil is almost colorless, having only a slight yellow tint. The inferior grades are greenish yellow. A very high-grade oil is also obtained by extracting the flowers with petroleum ether. This oil usually appears very dark.

Ilang-ilang oil is extensively used in the perfumery industry. It is employed in the preparation of high grade perfumes such as lily of the valley, corylopsis, etc.

Askinson † gives the formulas of various perfumes containing ilang-ilang as one of the principal constituents. The formula of one of these perfumes is as follows:

Heliotrope

Oil of ylang-ylang	drops....	20
Geraniol	do......	10
Benzaldehyde	do......	2
Heliotropin	grains....	35
Vanillin	do......	6
Coumarin	do......	4
Tincture of musk (xylene 100%)	do......	40
Cologne spirit (95%) enough to make	quart....	1

The manufacture of ilang-ilang oil is the most important, in fact, it is practically the only perfume industry in the Philippines. This oil is peculiarly a product of the Philippines. According to Parry ‡ oil distilled in other tropical countries from the same tree is not ranked in the same class as the Philippine product as regards quality. The value and amount of ilang-ilang exported from the Philippine Islands for the last four years are given in Table 30.

---

* Frequently spelled ylang-ylang.

† Askinson, G. W., Perfumes and cosmetics, (1915).

‡ Parry, E. J., Chemistry of essential oils and artificial perfumes, (1908).

TABLE 30.—*Amount and value of ilang-ilang oil exported from the Philippine Islands.*

Year.	Amount.	Value.
	Kilograms.	Pesos.
1915	1,277	43,514
1916	975	75,032
1917	2,286	93,951
1918	476	65,595

MANUFACTURE OF OIL

The flowers are usually picked at night and are collected in' the morning by the people who deliver them at the distilleries. In Manila the best flowers are usually obtained in May and June. We have little information as to the yield of flowers produced by a single tree, but it is apparently large.

Bacon,* who made an extensive investigation of ilang-ilang oil, did not believe that the distillation offered any special difficulties, but that it was necessary to collect only the proper fraction. He found that when the flowers are distilled commercially the procedure is frequently not carried out in the proper manner and that consequently a low grade of oil is often obtained.

* * * The important points where many err, and this is especially true of the provincial distillers, is in the wrong choice of fractions, in' burning the flowers and in obtaining too much resin in the oil. The oil must be distilled slowly, with *clean steam*, the flowers being so placed in the stills as to avoid their being cut into channels by the steam. The quantity of the oil taken is only a fraction of the total amount in the flowers. Disregard of this factor is one of the most grievous errors of the provincial distillers, for, on the contrary, they are usually too anxious to obtain a large yield of oil, and therefore they will often distill 1 kilo' from 150 to 200 kilos of flowers. The quantity of the latter to be taken to produce 1 kilo of oil naturally varies with their quality, but in general the amount should be 300 to 500 kilos, probably averaging about 400. After the first quality oil has been distilled, then a varying quantity of the second grade, up to a volume equal to that of the first, may be obtained from the same lot of flowers; after this operation the still and condensers must be thoroughly cleaned and steamed out to prevent contamination of

---

* Bacon, R. F., Philippine terpenes and essential oils, II. Ylang-ylang oil. Philippine Journal of Science, Section A, Volume 3 (1908), page 65.

Bacon, R. F., Philippine terpenes and essential oils, III. Oil of Ylang-ylang. Philippine Journal of Science, Section A, Volume 4 (1909), page 127.

Bacon, R. F., Philippine terpenes and essential oils, IV. Oil of Ylang-, ylang. Philippine Journal of Science, Section A, Volume 5 (1910), page 265.

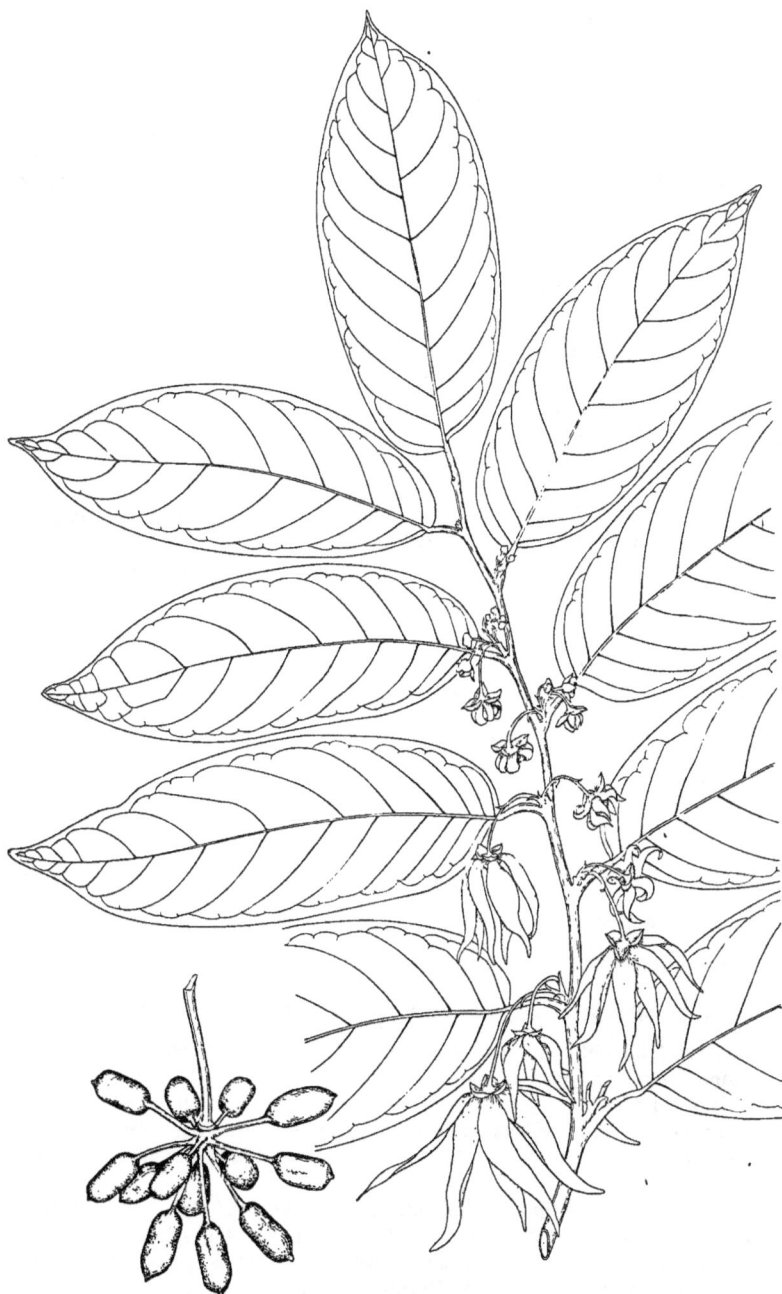

FIGURE 61. CANANGIUM ODORATUM (ILANG-ILANG), THE SOURCE OF ILANG-ILANG OIL. ×½.

the next distillation of first quality oil with the remains of the second quality adhering to the apparatus. The distiller usually judges of the time to change the receptacle from that used for first quality to that employed for the second, by taking note of the odor of the distillate. The oil is received in some type of Florence flask, usually two or more of these are connected in series and the condensed water is used in future distillations. The whole apparatus is best lined with block tin, although some distillers have found nickel to be more satisfactory. The oil, after separating from the water, is clarified and as it is sensitive to light and air, it should be placed into dark colored bottles as soon as possible; these should be filled to the neck, well stoppered and then paraffined to keep out all air. In the ideal apparatus the receivers should be so constructed that very little light and air has access to the oil. * * *

Bacon emphasized the fact that only mature, yellow flowers should be used, and he believed that the greatest advance in the industry would take place when the distillers owned their own groves and could select their flowers. This is shown very strikingly in the following quotation:

Fifty-four and five-tenths kilos (120 pounds) of extra fine flowers, one-half of which were perfectly yellow and ripe, were distilled with steam in the usual manner and the following fractions were obtained:

Number 1: 55 cubic centimeters; specific gravity, $\frac{30}{4}=0.960$;

$A\frac{30}{D}=-19.8°$; $N\frac{30}{D}=1.4865$; ester number, 178.

Number 2: 33 cubic centimeters; specific gravity, $\frac{30°}{4°}=0.959$;

$A\frac{30}{D}=-26.5°$; $N\frac{30°}{D}=1.4914$; ester number, 160.

Number 3: 90 cubic centimeters; specific gravity, $\frac{30}{4}=0.954$;

$A\frac{30°}{D}=-34.6°$; $N\frac{30°}{D}=1.4956$; ester number, 154.

Number 4: 80 cubic centimeters; specific gravity, $\frac{30°}{4}=0.942$;

$A\frac{30}{D}=-53.4°$; $N\frac{30}{D}=1.5020$; ester number, 113.

Tubes numbers 1, 2 and 3 united gave the following constants: Specific gravity, $\frac{30°}{4}=0.958$; $A\frac{30°}{D}=-27.0$; $N\frac{30°}{D}=1.4910$; ester number, 169.

The total oil obtained was 258 cubic centimeters, which is 264 grams, corresponding to a yield of 0.45 per cent.

This yield was nearly twice the normal amount and the quality of the oil was very high, as was shown not only by analytical figures given above, but also was confirmed by the opinions of Manila experts to whom it was submitted.

I believe these experiments indicate that 200 kilos of ripe, yellow flowers will give 1 kilo of a better quality of oil than will 400 kilos of the class of poor, mixed flowers used at the present time. It is a well-known fact of plant physiology that the odoriferous substance is present in the flowers in greatest abundance and in finest quality at the time when it is mature

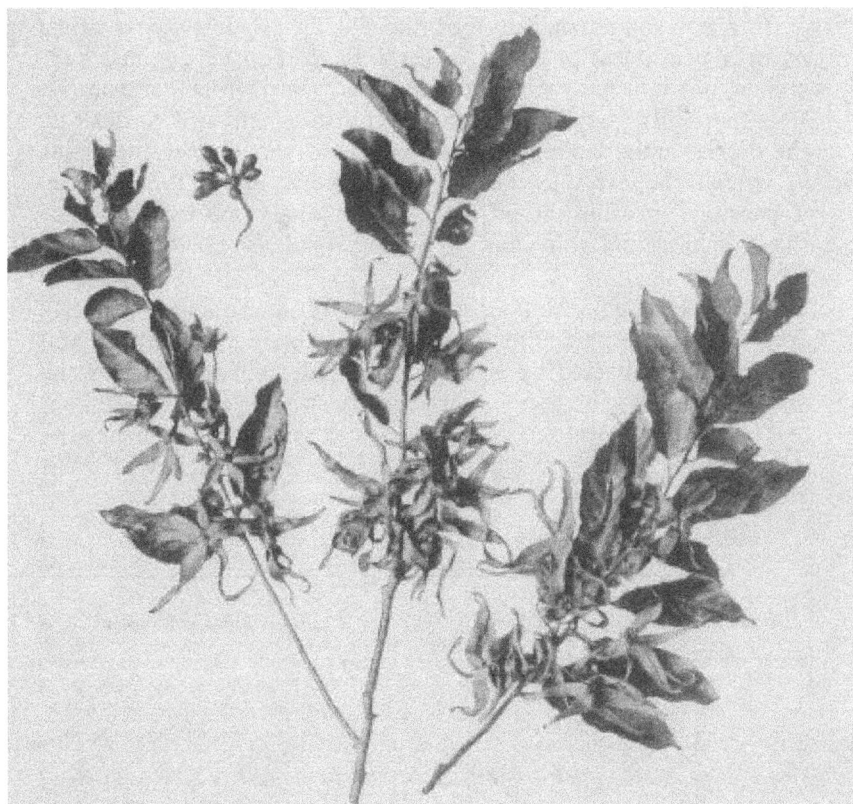

FIGURE 62. CANANGIUM ODORATUM (ILANG-ILANG), THE SOURCE OF ILANG-ILANG OIL.

and ready for pollination. No doubt, in the course of time much can be done toward improving the yield and quality of ilang-ilang oil by intelligent plant selection. Such work requires much patience and at present there are absolutely no data available save a general opinion that the ilang-ilang trees of the wild mountain regions are not as fragrant as the cultivated ones of the lowlands.

CLASSIFICATION OF ILANG-ILANG OIL

It is a well-known fact that ilang-ilang oil, like many other natural perfumes, does not owe its fragrance to any one substance, but is a mixture of a number of odoriferous compounds. It is generally bought and sold on the judgment of the dealers, the determining factor being the odor. Obviously the judgment of various buyers may differ, and consequently it is desirable, if possible, to value the oil according to analytical tests, so that the purchase and sale may be placed upon an exact analytical basis.

Bacon obtained a number of samples of ilang-ilang oil, mostly from one distillery, the process of distillation being watched and the samples collected by himself. He determined a few of the simple constants of these oils, such as specific gravity (pyknometer), optical rotation, refractive index, and ester number; the latter by the usual method, using 1 gram of oil. A few of these results are recorded in Table 31.

TABLE 31.—*Tabulation of the constants of ilang-ilang oils.*

Grade.	Sample.	Sp. gr. $\frac{30^{\circ}}{4^{\circ}}$.	$a\ \frac{30^{\circ}}{D}$.	$n\ \frac{30^{\circ}}{D}$.	Ester number.	Origin and remarks.
First	5	0.939	−34.2	1.4880	131	B.'s distillate of August 22, 1907.
	10	0.922	−26.0	1.4794	117	First quality oil rectified *in vacuo*. B.'s distillate 90 per cent yield.
	21	0.949	−36.1	1.4940	138	Distilled *in vacuo* with steam from selected flowers.
	22	0.827	−42.2	1.4912	126	B.'s distillate of Febuary 1, 1908, from very good flowers.
	23	0.958	−27.0	1.4910	169	0.4 per cent yield from selected flowers with very careful distillation. A very fine oil.
Second	12	0.917	−66.7	1.5032	70	Distillation of second-quality oil from flowers from which the first quality had been previously distilled. Yield, 0.7 per cent.
	13	0.919	−61.4	1.4977	86	Second-quality oil.
	14	0.918	−66.4	1.4986	83	Second-quality oil.
	15	0.903	−81.3	1.4981	59	Second-quality oil.
	16	0.928	−30.2	1.4927	64	Provincial oil.

The determination of these constants enables us to classify oils into first and second grades. The limits for these grades are given in Table 32.

TABLE 32.—*Classification of ilang-ilang oil according to Bacon.*

Constants.	First grade.	Second grade.
Ester number	100 and above	80 to 100.
Index of refraction	1.4900 and below	Above 1.4900.
Specific rotation	−45° and below	Above−45°.

In a later publication Bacon showed that first-grade oils have a higher acetyl number than second-grade oils.

The classification of ilang-ilang oil now in use is a modification of Bacon's standard of classification, which was proposed by Dr. Jaehrling of the firm of Santos and Jaehrling of Manila, and advocated by Gibbs.* The constants of this classification are given in Table 33. This classification divides Bacon's first class into three divisions, namely: extra, 1–a, and 1–b. This division is apparently necessary on account of the large proportion of high-grade oil which is now produced.

TABLE 33.—*Classification of ilang-ilang oil according to Jaehrling.*

Grade.	Ester number.	Index of refraction.	Specific rotation.	Solubility in alcohol of—
				Per cent.
Extra	Above 145	Below 1.4900	Above−35	80.
1a	120 to 145	1.4900 to 1.4950	−35 to—48	90.
1b	100 to 120	1.4950 to 1.4990	−48 to—60	90-96.
2	Below 100	Above 1.4990	Below—60	96

The solubility of ilang-ilang in alcohol is also given as an extra test. According to Gibbs, this is very useful as a confirmatory test, since it indicates the amount of sesquiterpenes present in the oil. This test consists in determining the lowest strength of aqueous alcohol which can be mixed with the oil without cloudiness, in the proportion of 2 of oil to 1 of alcohol.

Bacon suggests an easy method of judging approximately the quality of an oil:

---

* Gibbs, H. D., Proposed modification of ilang-ilang oil standards. Philippine Journal of Science, Section A, Volume 10 (1915), page 99.

* * * To prepare a 1 per cent solution of the oil in alcohol and
compare the odor with a similar one of an oil of known quality, as judgment is much more certain as to the perfuming power when dilute solutions
instead of the pure oils are used. One cubic centimeter of each solution
can then be poured on separated pieces of bibulous paper, the odor being
compared at the end of twelve, twenty-four, or even a longer number of
hours; this test gives some idea in regard to the permanence of the odor.

DISTILLATION OF OIL IN VACUO

Bacon found that the distillation of the oil *in vacuo* provides
a good method of ascertaining the quality of an oil and the number of flowers used in preparing it. He also showed that the
rectification of oils *in vacuo* is not very successful. These points
are shown in the following quotation:

* * * the rectification of oils *in vacuo* is not an entire success, as
the distillates, although apparently of the same composition as the oil
from which they are distilled, seem to lack in perfuming power; this is
especially true of the lasting qualities of the odor. These results suggest
that the highest boiling parts of the ilang-ilang oil and even the resins,
are very probably important constituents of the whole, possibly they help
to fix the more volatile, odoriferous portions. I have always been im-
pressed by the peculiarly lasting fragrance of the resinous residues of the
distillation of ilang-ilang oils fractioned *in vacuo*.

The distillation of ilang-ilang oils *in vacuo* has shown that over 50 per
cent of the first quality oil will pass over below 100° at 10 millimeters
pressure, and when I have tested poorer oils in this respect I have found
the amount of substance volatile below 100° at 10 millimeters which
passed over to be proportional to the quantity of flowers used in preparing
the oil. Thus one oil distilled from flowers at the yield of 1 kilo for 206
kilos of flowers showed 27 per cent of volatile constituents under the conditions named, whereas another prepared in the proportion of 1 kilo to
150 kilos of flowers gave 19 per cent.

It follows from this that the distillation test is also of value both in
determining the quality of an oil and the proportion of flowers used in
preparing it. The only manner in which poor provincial oils may be
improved is by redistillation with steam, and this procedure results in
large losses. Fractioning with steam *in vacuo* also seems quite promising,
although the process is very slow. Oils thus obtained are quite colorless,
and by taking suitable fractions a very fair oil may thus be prepared from
a product which before treatment was almost unsalable.

EXTRACTION OF PERFUME OIL WITH SOLVENTS

Bacon * also studied the problem of extracting the oil from
ilang-ilang flowers with solvents:

* * * Many of the constituents of essential oils are very delicate
substances and distillation with steam decomposes these compounds to a

---

* Bacon, R. F., Philippine terpenes and essential oils, III. Philippine
Journal of Science, Section A, Volume 4 (1909), page 129.

considerable extent, so that a steam-distilled oil but rarely has exactly the same odor as the flowers from which it was obtained. Extraction with cold solvents and the removal of the solvent *in vacuo*, the temperature never being allowed to rise above 40°, gives oils which have exactly the same aroma as the flowers. This process has the further commercial advantage that such extracted flower oils can not be imitated synthetically, as the change in aroma is undoubtedly due to traces of very easily decomposable compounds which it will be difficult, if not impossible, ever to isolate and identify. The extracted oil need fear no competition with synthetic oils. Alcohol, ether, chloroform and petroleum ether have been used as solvents for ilang-ilang oil, and the last named has given the best results. Naturally, a very high grade of petroleum ether, which leaves no bad smelling residue when distilled up to 40° in a vacuum of 40 millimeters, must be used as the solvent for the essential oil. Operating in this manner, we have obtained oil yields of from 0.7 to 1.0 per cent. The oil is of a very dark color and contains a considerable amount of resin in solution. When in bulk, the odor is not particularly pleasant or very strong, but when the extract is greatly diluted the pleasant aroma of the flowers becomes very apparent. The physical constants of one sample of this oil were as follows: Specific gravity, $\frac{30°}{4°} = 0.940$; N $\frac{30°}{D} = 1.4920$; ester number 135; acetyl number 208.

The oil is too dark to permit readings of its optical rotation to be practicable. These constants are seen to agree quite well with those of a very high grade distilled oil, and as was stated above, the different odor is probably due to traces of delicate compounds present in the extracted oil, which are destroyed during the process of distillation. It is rather curious to note that when this extracted oil is shaken out with water, a considerable amount of resin separates, carrying the distinctive flower aroma, and the separated oil then has an odor resembling that of methyl-*p*-kresol.

These extracted oils should sell for a considerably higher price than the best distilled oils, which fact, taken in consideration with the increased yield and the impossibility of competition from synthetic oils, offers a very . attractive new industry to the Philippines.

ADULTERANTS

Regarding the use of adulterants of ilang-ilang oil, Bacon says that he does not believe the practice is very general in the Philippines. The common adulterants are said to be turpentine, coconut or other fixed oils, and kerosene. Bacon suggests various tests for these substances, if their presence is suspected.*

The use of any adulteration is more emphatically the height of commercial folly for ilang-ilang than it is for any other essential oil, for only the product of the highest quality brings a remunerative price. A 10 per cent increase in quantity by means of adulteration may cut the price in two, or may result in an oil which can not be sold at any price. * * *

---

* Bacon, R. F., Philippine terpenes and essential oils, II. Ylang-ylang oil. Philippine Journal of Science, Section A, Volume 3 (1908), page 76.

COMPOSITION OF ILANG-ILANG OIL

Parry states that investigations of ilang-ilang oil have shown that it contains esters of benzoic and acetic acids, also linaloöl, cadinene, pinene, P-cresol methyl ether, geraniol, and iso-eugenol. Parry is of the opinion that in addition to these substances, ilang-ilang contains other compounds, as a synthetic oil closely resembling the natural oil has been prepared commercially. Probably a considerable amount of research has been done on ilang-ilang, but for trade reasons the investigators do not care to publish their results.

Bacon * performed a number of experiments to determine the composition of ilang-ilang oil and concluded that it contained ' formic, acetic, valerianic (?), benzoic, and salicylic acids, all as esters; methyl and benzyl alcohols; pinene and other terpenes, linaloöl, geraniol, safrol, cadinene and other sesquiterpenes; eugenol, iso-eugenol, p-cresol, probably as methyl ethers; and cresol. He then prepared a synthetic oil in order to test the accuracy of his studies on the composition of ilang-ilang oil. His synthetic ilang-ilang contained the following substances (proportions not stated): methyl benzoate; benzyl acetate and formate; benzyl methyl ether (trace); benzyl valerianate (trace); methyl salicylate; benzyl benzoate; cadinene; safrol; iso-eugenol-methyl ether; eugenol; cresol; methyl anthranilate (trace); p-cresol-methyl ether; p-cresol acetate. This mixture ' gave an odor very similar to good ilang-ilang oil. From the results of his own work and that of others Bacon concluded:

* * * ylang-ylang oil has a composite odor, derived from that of many constituents. While it is possible to make a very good artificial ylang-ylang oil, I do not believe that distillers of the best quality of ylang-ylang oil have much to fear from this competition, as the odor of a first-c class oil seems to have more permanence than that of the artificial product. This is a result, I believe, of the presence of sesquiterpene alcohols and fragrant resins in the former.

GROWTH OF CANANGIUM ODORATUM

This species has been grown in plantations at Los Baños. Only one lot of seeds was planted, and this showed a very low percentage of germination, 3.2 per cent. It is uncertain as to whether or not this low percentage was due to poor seed. The trees have done well in plantations. The average rates of growth of considerable numbers are given in Table 34.

---

* Bacon, R. F., Philippine terpenes and essential oils, II. Ylang-ylang (oil. Philippine Journal of Science, Section A, Volume 3 (1908), page 86.

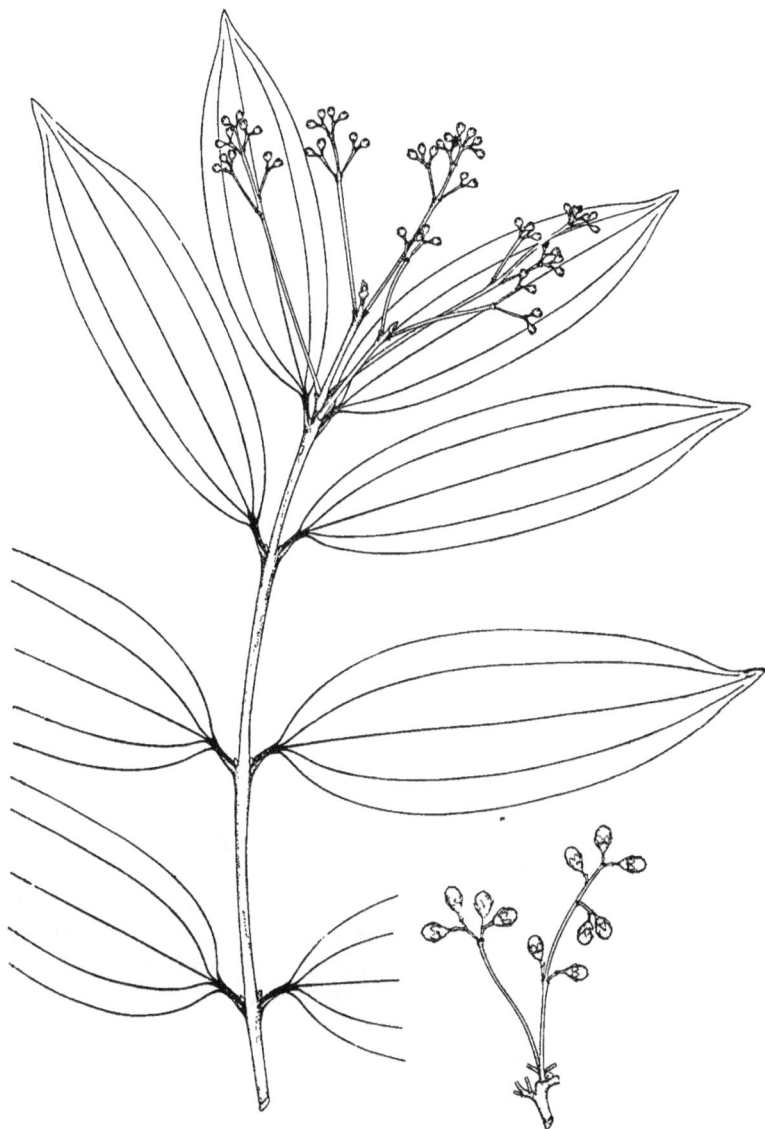

FIGURE 63. CINNAMOMUM INERS, A SOURCE OF CINNAMON. ×½.

TABLE 34.—*Growth of Canangium odoratum (Ilang-ilang) in plantations at Los Baños, Laguna.*

Age.	Diam-eter.	Height.
Years.	*cm.*	*m.*
2		1.33
3		2.05
4		3.80
5	7	5.34
7	12	8.35

Canangium odoratum is a medium-sized to rather large tree, with somewhat drooping branches. The leaves are alternate, 12 to 20 centimeters long, pointed at the apex, and usually rounded at the base. The flowers are very fragrant, greenish, soon turning yellowish, pendulous. The pedicels are 1 to 2.5 centimeters long and elongated in fruit. The sepals are hairy. The petals are somewhat hairy, narrow, pointed, 4 to 6 centimeters long and 0.5 to 1 centimeter wide.

This species is a native of the Philippines and is found throughout the Archipelago both cultivated and wild. It occurs at elevations of at least 700 meters. It is very commonly cultivated in Manila and flowers throughout the year.

Family LAURACEAE

Genus CINNAMOMUM

CINNAMOMUM INERS Reinw. (Fig. 63).   CINNAMON.

Local names: *Marobo* (Samar).

CINNAMON

The bark of this species is sold commercially as cinnamon. *Cinnamomum iners* is a small to large tree. The leaves are opposite, smooth, leathery, from 8 to 16 centimeters long, pointed at the apex and rounded or pointed at the base. The flowers are yellowish, about 4 millimeters long, and borne on compound inflorescences. The fruits are about a centimeter long.

This species has been reported from Mindoro, Palawan, Samar, Mindanao, and Tawi-tawi.

CINNAMOMUM MERCADOI Vid. (Fig. 64).   KALÍÑGAG.

Local names: *Canela* (Span. in Pangasinan); *kalíñgag* (Rizal, Bataan, Lanao, Laguna, Samar, Tayabas, Camarines, Polillo, Pampanga); *kalíñgad* (Pampanga); *kaníla* (Lepanto, Albay); *kanilao, kaníñgai* (Camarines); *kandaróma* (Benguet); *kasíu* (Calayan Island); *kulíuan* or *ulíuan* (Cagayan); *samíling* (Bataan).

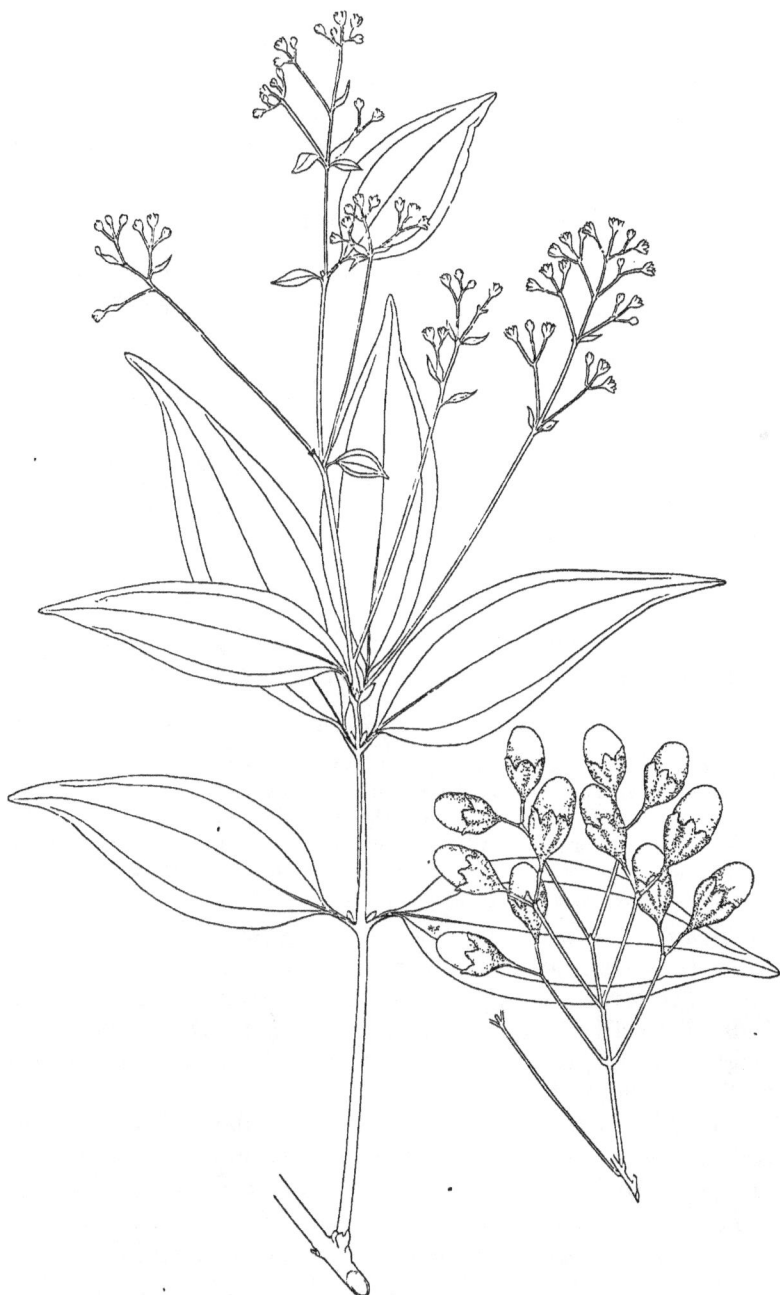

FIGURE 64. CINNAMOMUM MERCADOI (KALIÑGAG), THE SOURCE OF KALIÑGAG OIL.
X⅖.

KALIÑGAG OIL

The bark of *Cinnamomum mercadoi* is used locally as medicine and would probably, on account of its strong sassafras odor and taste, make a good ingredient for root beers.

Bacon * made a chemical investigation of this bark and reported his results as follows:

* * * I obtained 25 kilos of bark from the Lamao region, Bataan Province. This bark was ground and distilled with steam, giving 260 grams (1.04 per cent) of a light yellow oil. The oil had an odor like sassafras and the following properties: Specific gravity $\frac{30°}{4°}$=1.0461; $N\frac{30°}{D}$=1.5270; $A\frac{30°}{D}=+4°$. * * *

The oil was distilled at 10 millimeters and gave the following fractions:

No.	Boiling point.	Quantity.	$N\frac{30°}{D.}$
	Degrees.	*Grams.*	
1	119-124	77°	1.5333
2	124-130	9.2	1.5320
3	Residue	11.5	1.5278

Fraction No. 1 redistilled at ordinary pressure had a boiling point 235° to 238° at 760 millimeters; specific gravity, $\frac{30°}{4}$ =1.0631; $N\frac{30°}{D}$=1.5335; $A\frac{30°}{D}$ =+0.9. By oxidation with chromic acid this fraction gives piperonylic acid melting at 227°. Piperonal was obtained by heating with alcoholic potash and then oxidizing with potassium permanganate. These results leave no doubt but that the oil from *Cinnamomum mercadoi* Vid. is almost entirely safrol, and it is remarkable in this respect, as most oils from *Cinnamomum* species contain only small amounts of safrol and large percentages of cinnamic aldehyde. * * *

Cinnamomum mercadoi is a small to medium-sized tree up to 65 centimeters in diameter. It is usually straight but not very tall. The leaves are opposite, smooth, leathery, pointed at both ends, distinctly three-nerved, and from 8 to 20 centimeters in length. The fruits are about 2 centimeters long and surrounded to the middle by the persistent calyx.

This species is very widely distributed and well known, but rather scarce. Quantities of bark sufficient for commercial utilization could be collected, if it were of sufficient value.

CINNAMOMUM MINDANAENSE Elm. (Fig. 65). MINDANAO CINNAMON.

Local names: *Kaliñgag* (Surigao); *canela* (Span. in Zamboanga).

---

* Bacon, R. F., Philippine terpenes and essential oils, III. Philippine Journal of Science, Section A, Volume 4 (1909), page 114.

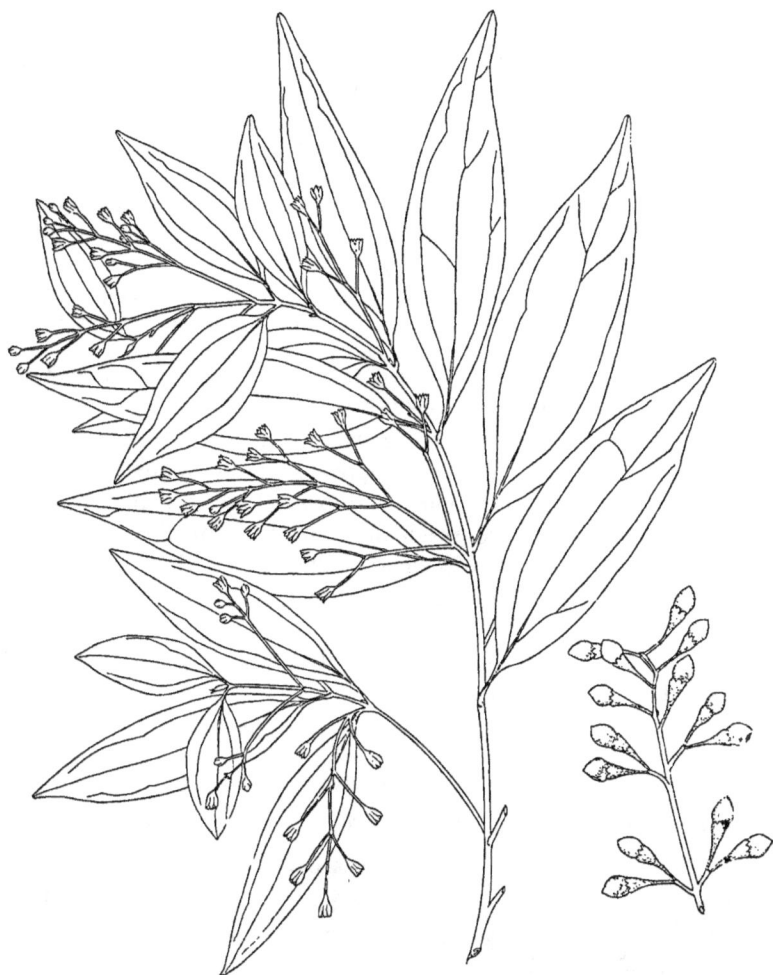

FIGURE 65. CINNAMOMUM MINDANAENSE (MINDANAO CINNAMON), A SOURCE OF
CINNAMON. $\times\frac{1}{2}$.

CINNAMON

The bark of this species is collected and sold as cinnamon of commerce.

Bacon * examined the bark, and reported as follows:

* * * The tree is very close to *Cinnamomum zeylanicum* Nees and the bark in appearance, taste, and odor is just like the cinnamon of commerce. Fifty kilos of the ground bark were distilled with steam, yielding 200 grams of oil of a yellow color and of a strong cinnamon odor and taste.

This probably does not represent by any means all of the oil which it is possible to obtain by commercial distillation from this bark, the proportion being less because of the small amount of material at my disposal. The oil had the following properties: Refractive index, $N\frac{30°}{D}$ 1.5300; optical rotation, $A\frac{30'}{D}$ 7°.9; specific gravity, $\frac{30}{30}$ 0.960.

Ten grams of the oil gave 9.2 grams of the dry sodium bisulphite compound of cinnamic aldehyde, corresponding to an aldehyde content of approximately 60 per cent.

This oil does not agree very closely in its physical properties with the Ceylon cinnamon oil from *C. zeylanicum*.

Cinnamomum mindanaense is usually a small tree, about 10 meters in height. The leaves are opposite or sub-opposite, smooth, leathery, pointed at both ends, and from 7 to 15 centimeters in length. The flowers are greenish, about 5 millimeters long, and borne on compound inflorescences. The fruits when mature are shining steel-blue, 1.25 centimeters long, and 7.5 millimeters in width.

This species is known only from Mindanao, where it is fairly abundant in some places.

Family LEGUMINOSAE

Genus ACACIA

ACACIA FARNESIANA Willd. (Fig. 66).   CASSIE FLOWER or AROMA.

CASSIE-FLOWER OIL

A gum which resembles gum arabic exudes from the bark of this tree. The flowers are known commercially as cassie flowers. *Acacia farnesiana* is grown extensively in France for the fragrant perfume obtained from the flowers. The odor of this perfume resembles that of violets, but is more intense. Piesse † states that cassie perfume is one of those fine odors which are

---

* Bacon, R. F., Philippine terpenes and essential oils, IV. Philippine Journal of Science, Section A, Volume 5 (1910), page 257.

† Piesse, C. H., Art of perfumery, (1891).

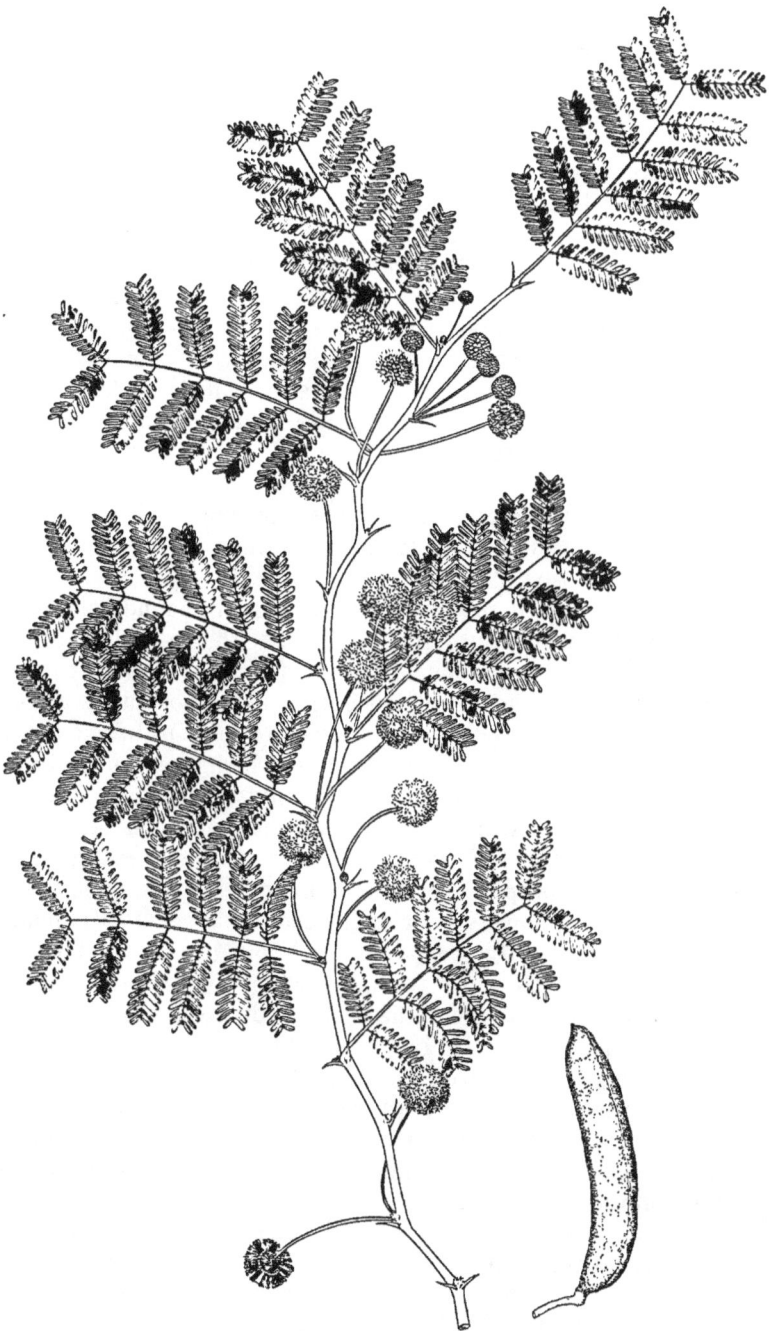

FIGURE 66. ACACIA FARNESIANA (AROMA), THE SOURCE OF CASSIE FLOWERS. ×½.

used in preparing the best handkerchief bouquets and hair pomades. When diluted with other odors it imparts to the whole a true flowery fragrance.

The essential oil obtained from the flowers of *Acacia farnesia* is greenish yellow and viscid. This oil itself is never sold commercially, but is mixed with other substances and sold as perfumes, fixed oils, pomades, or extract of cassie.

Cassie perfume is prepared as a pomade by macerating the flower heads and placing the crushed material in purified melted fat where it is allowed to remain several hours. As many flowers are used as the fluid grease will cover. The spent flowers are next removed and replaced by fresh ones. This operation is continued until the grease has acquired a sufficient richness of perfume. Eight or ten treatments are usually necessary. The melted fat is then strained and cooled. This preparation, which is simply a solution of the true essential oil of cassie flowers in a neutral fat, is the commercial cassie pomade. More modern methods of preparing pomades such as that of cassie are described by Askinson.*

Extract of cassie is prepared by treating six pounds of cassie pomade, which is cut into small pieces, with one gallon of alcohol. Askinson * uses four pounds of cassie pomade to one gallon of alcohol. The alcoholic solution of the pomade is placed in securely stoppered bottles and allowed to remain three or four weeks at summer heat. The perfume which the fat contains is dissolved out by the alcohol. The mixture is then filtered. The residue of fat still contains some perfume and serves as an excellent material for the manufacture of hair dressing. The extract of cassie prepared in this manner has a fine olive-green color and the rich flowery odor of the cassie blossoms. It should be preserved in tightly stoppered bottles in a cool, dark place. This is necessary, as under the influence of light, heat, and air, the delightful odors of perfumes are gradually destroyed.

Cassie perfume may also be prepared by distilling the flowers and dissolving the essential oil thus obtained in alcohol. This method of preparation gives, however, an inferior product, which does not have the true, natural scent of the flowers. Usually, when the active odorous principle of the flower exists in unusually minute quantities as in such flowers as cassie, violet, and jasmine, a better grade of perfume is obtained by making a pomade, rather than by distilling.

* Askinson, G. W., Perfumes and cosmetics, (1915).

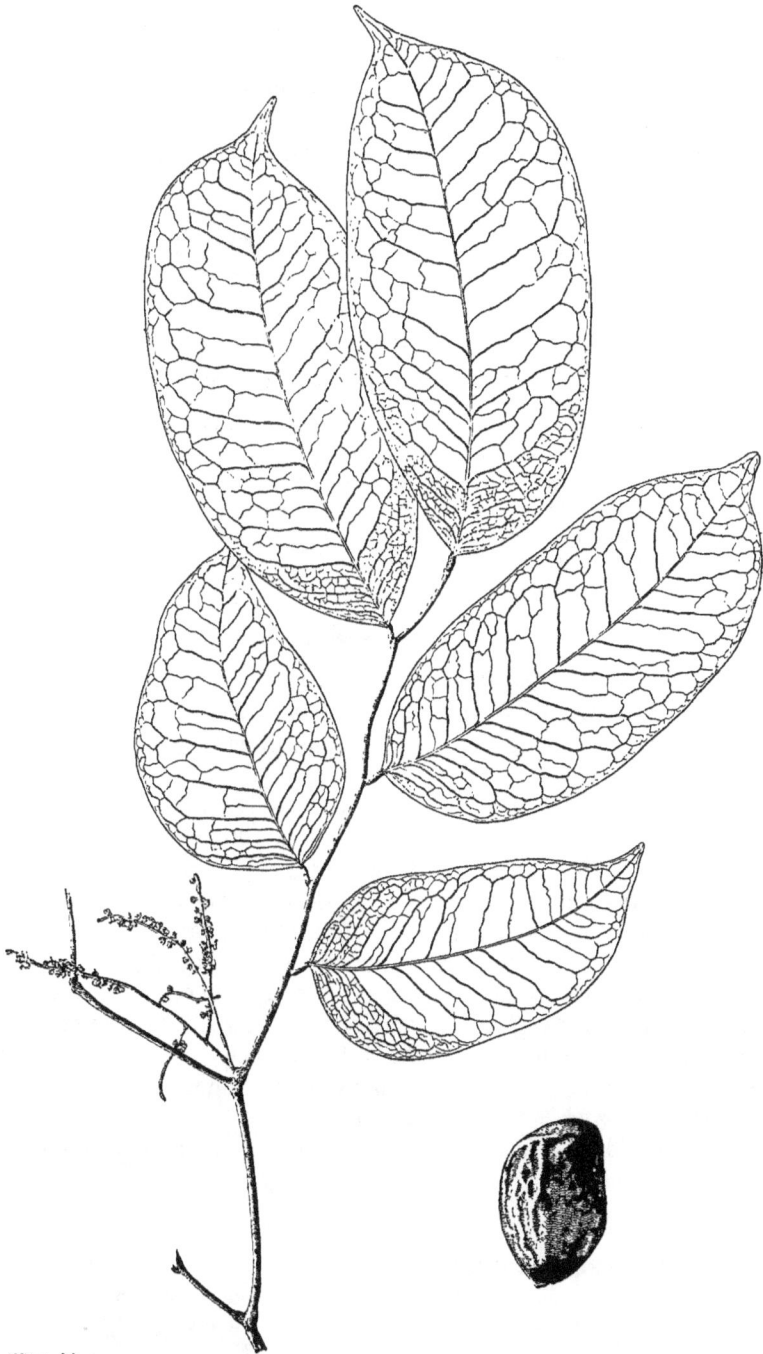

JVitan del.

FIGURE 67. KINGIODENDRON ALTERNIFOLIUM (BATÉTE), THE SOURCE OF BATÉTE INCENSE.

Acacia farnesiana is a large, spiny shrub or small tree from 3 to 4 meters in height. The leaves are 5 to 8 centimeters long, and bipinnate, usually with ten to twelve leaflets. The leaflets are 4 to 7 millimeters in length. The flowers are yellow and fragrant and are borne in dense, globose heads, which are about 1 centimeter in diameter. The pods are 5 to 7 centimeters long and 1 to 1.5 centimeters wide, straight or curved. This species is probably a native of tropical America, but is widely distributed in waste places in the Philippines and is one of the commonest plants in the early stages of the invasion of grasslands by second-growth forests.

Genus KINGIODENDRON

KINGIODENDRON ALTERNIFOLIUM Merr.   (Figs. 67, 68).   BATÉTE.

Local names: *Batéte* (Tayabas, Sorsogon, Ticao Island, Masbate); *danggái* (Camarines, Tayabas, Albay, Sorsogon, Masbate); *duká* (Negros, Tablas Island, Leyte); *kalikít* (Agusan); *kumagasáka, paliná* (Agusan, Davao); *longbayau* or *manogbayo* (Agusan); *bagbalógo, magabalogo* (Samar); *palomaría* (Zamboanga); *salaláñgin* (Albay, Sorsogon); *sarok* (Davao); *painá, pariná* or *payiná* (Camarines, Albay, Sorsogon); *tuá-an* (Misamis).

BATÉTE INCENSE

Batete has a dark-green sap which thickens to a gummy consistency on exposure. Nothing is known of its chemical properties, but mention is made in Spanish literature of its use for incense.

Kingiodendron alternifolium is a tree reaching a height of 30 to 35 meters and a diameter of 80 to 100 centimeters. The bark is 7 to 10 millimeters thick, gray to gray brown with a yellowish tinge, and is shed in large scroll-shaped patches. The inner bark is red. The leaves are alternate, and simply compound with from 3 to 7, usually alternate, leaflets, which are smooth, leathery, pointed at the apex, rounded or pointed at the base, and from 8 to 18 centimeters long. The flowers are small and borne on compound inflorescences. The fruits are rounded or oval, frequently somewhat flattened, 4 to 5 centimeters long, and 3 to 4 centimeters wide. This species is distributed from central Luzon to Mindanao.

Family RUTACEAE

Genus CITRUS

CITRUS HYSTRIX DC. (Fig. 69).   KABÚYAU.

Local names: *Duñgaruñgut* (Cagayan); *kabúyau* (Pampanga, Tarlac, Bulacan, Zambales, Bataan, Manila, Batangas, Laguna, Zamboanga);

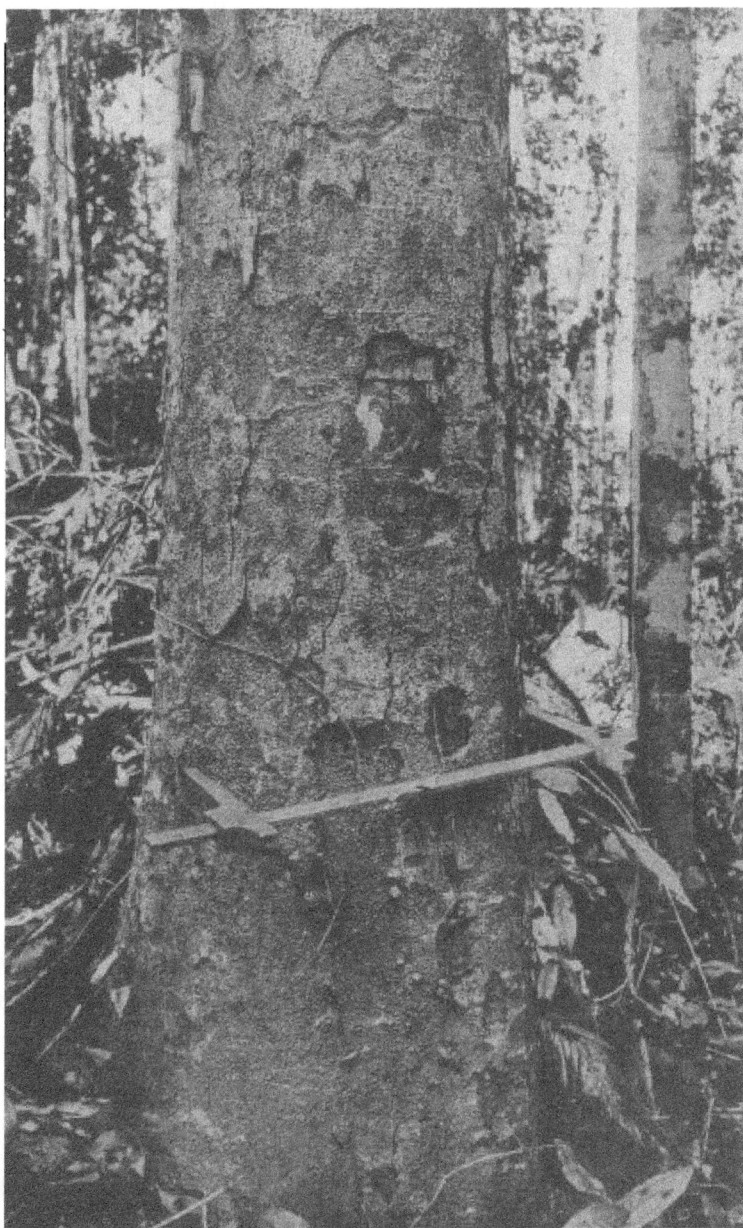

FIGURE 68. TRUNK OF KINGIODENDRON ALTERNIFOLIUM (BATÉTE), THE SOURCE OF BATÉTE INCENSE.

kabúgau (Camarines, Mindoro); *kamúlau* (Iloko); *kamuntai* (Bisaya);ᶜ
kamúyau (Ilocos Norte and Sur, Abra); *kapítan* (Iloko); *kolobót* (Tagalog); *limón-karabáu* (Zamboanga); *makatbá* (Zambales); *peres* (Pangasinan).

KABÚYAU OIL

Schimmel * states that the oil of this species has an odor
resembling that of bergamot. According to Brooks,† the leaves
of the Philippine plant when steam-distilled yield an oil resembling in odor the oil distilled from the leaves of the pomelo,
Citrus decumana Murr. Although the oil is very fragrant, the
yield (0.08 per cent) is extremely small. The constants of the
oil are as follows: Specific gravity, $\frac{30°}{30}$ =0.9150; N $\frac{30}{D}$ =1.4650;
A $\frac{30}{D}$ = −10.50°; saponification number, 50.2.

Citrus hystrix is a small tree armed with small spines. The
leaves are variable, but average 10 to 12 centimeters in length.
The flowers are white and about a centimeter wide. The fruits
are about 10 centimeters in diameter.

This species is common and widely distributed in forests
throughout the Philippines.

CITRUS MICRANTHA var. MICROCARPA Wester. (Fig. 70). SAMÚYAU.

SAMÚYAU OIL

The rind of this species yields a clear, almost colorless oil
which is very fragrant. It should be useful as a perfumery
oil.

The crushed fruits or samúyau are used by women in Cebu
for cleansing the hair, or are mixed with Gogo (pounded stems
of *Entada phaseoloides*) which serves as a shampoo. The
crushed fruit is also added to coconut oil, to give it fragrance
when applied to the hair.

The oil obtained by steam-distilling the crushed peels had an
orange-like odor and the following constants:

Specific gravity	28.5°=	0.8670
Refractive index	25°=	1.4718.
Optical rotation	A $\frac{30}{D}$ =	−1.150
(100 mm. tube)		

---

* Schimmel, Semi-annual report (1901).

† Brooks, B. T., New Philippine essential oils. Philippine Journal of
Science, Section A, Volume 6 (1911), page 349.

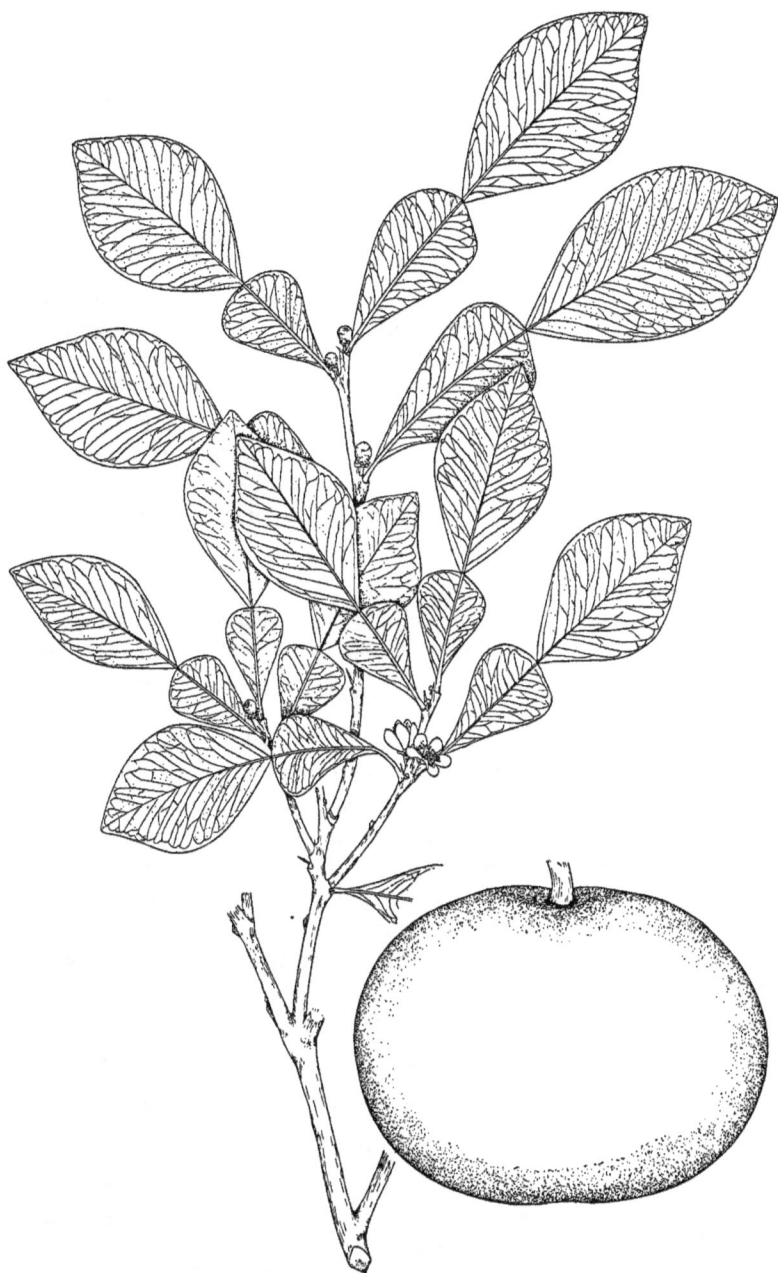

FIGURE 69. CITRUS HYSTRIX (KABÚYAU), THE SOURCE OF KABÚYAU OIL. ×½.

The yield of oil, calculated from the weight of the whole fruit, was 0.56 per cent and from the peel alone 1.29 per cent. The oil has been employed as an ingredient of shampoos. The tree is said to bear fruits within five years after planting. The fruits are produced during the entire year, but most abundantly during the rainy season. In places where they are grown they sell for 5 centavos per hundred during the wet and 20 centavos per hundred during the dry season. Samuyau is said to be very delicate, and to need careful attention, and in Cebu, during the dry season, even daily watering.

Citrus micrantha var. *microcarpa* is a shrubby tree about 4.5 meters tall. It has slender branches and small, weak spines. The leaves are thin, with a distinct fragrance, 5.5 to 8 centimeters long, and 2 to 2.5 centimeters broad. The flowers are white with a trace of purple on the outside, and 5 to 9 millimeters in diameter. The fruit is 1.5 to 2 centimeters in diameter, roundish in outline, and greenish lemon-yellow.

This species is abundant in Cebu and other islands of the Bisaya group.

CITRUS Sp.   GURONG-GURÓ.

Local names: *Bungkalót* (Laguna); *kabúrau* (Iloko); *kolison, muntai* (Tayabas); *gurong-guró* (Pangasinan, Zambales); *suangi* (Manila); *tibulíd* (Bulacan).

GURONG-GURO

This species has a very fragrant rind which is mixed with coconut oil for use on the hair. The whole fruit is also mixed with gogo (*Entada phaseoloides*) bark as a shampoo. Cloves are sometimes put into the rind and then the fruits squeezed in the hands to give them a pleasant odor. The fruit of this species is about 5 centimeters in diameter, with a very rough, irregularly ridged, green rind, and with a nipple-like protuberance at the base. The rind is rather thin, and the fruit is not edible.

Genus CLAUSENA

CLAUSENA ANISUM-OLENS (Blanco) Merr. (Fig. 71).   KAYUMANÍS.

Local names: *Dayap-dayápan* (Laguna); *kayumanís* (Rizal).

CLAUSENA ANISUM-OLENS OIL

The leaves have an odor much like that of anise. Bacon * says that alcoholic extracts also have a very strong anise-like odor. According to him, it is possible that this plant could be used

---

* Bacon, R. F., Philippine terpenes and essential oils, III. Philippine Journal of Science, Section A, Volume 4 (1909), page 130.

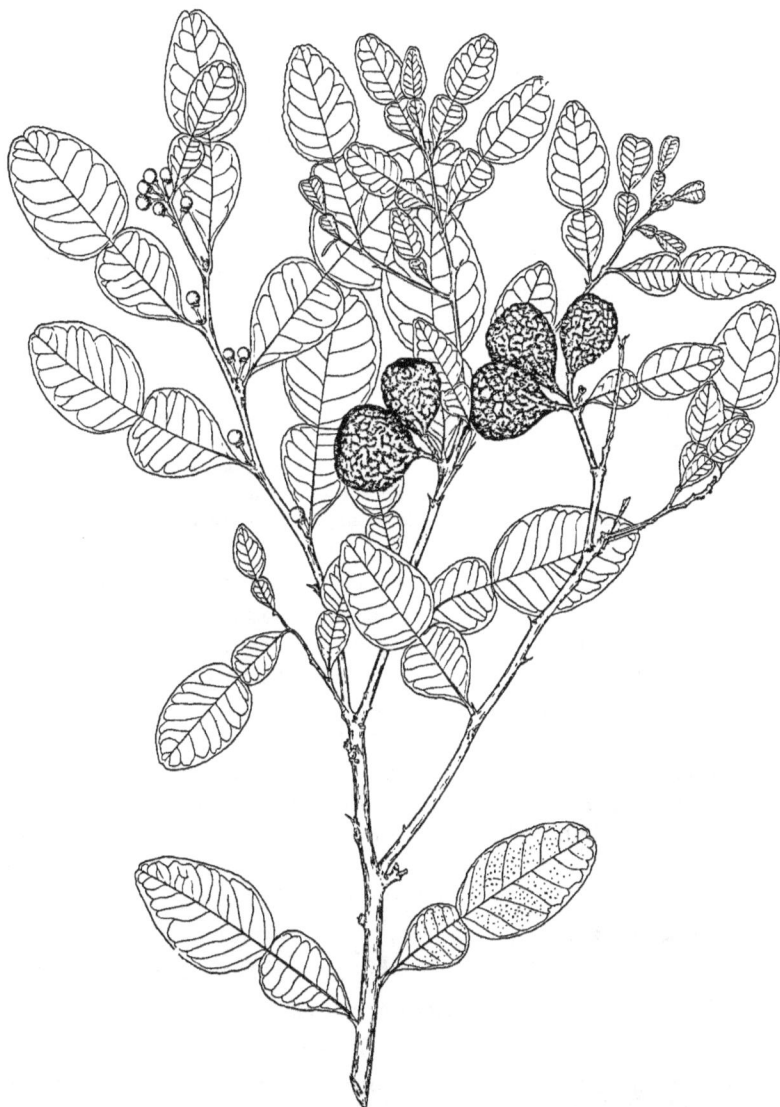

FIGURE 70. CITRUS MICRANTHA VAR. MICROCARPA (SAMÚYAU), THE SOURCE OF
SAMÚYAU OIL. ×⅜.

locally in preparing anisado, which is a favorite alcoholic beverage among the Filipinos.

Brooks * examined the oil obtained from the leaves of this species and states that:

A quantity of leaves, weighing approximately 16 kilos, were distilled with steam over a period of about five hours and 185 grams of colorless oil were obtained. This oil resembled the fresh leaves in odor and possessed the following constants. Specific gravity, $\frac{30}{30°} = 0.963$; N $\frac{30°}{D} = 1.5235$; saponification number 3.6; the oil is inactive. * * *

The oil has a faint odor of anise or anethol, which, together with the constants, identifies it almost with certainty as methyl chavicol. For further proof, a small portion was oxidized with potassium permanganate to homoanisic acid, melting point, 84° to 86°. * * *

Therefore, it is evident that the oil from *Clausena* contains methyl chavicol to the extent of 90 to 95 per cent. * * *

The occurrence of methyl chavicol, especially in such large proportions, in one of the *Rutaceae* is quite novel. * * *

Owing to the ease with which methyl chavicol is converted into anethol, by treatment with alkalies, it is possible that this operation would be successful commercially. Considerable quantities of anise oil are annually imported into the Philippine Islands for the manufacture of *anisado*. However it is doubtful whether or not *Clausena* could successfully be cultivated, as it is a typical forest species.

Clausena anisum-olens is a small tree, 3 to 6 meters high. The leaves are alternate, 20 to 30 centimeters long, compound, with 7 to 11 leaflets which are inequilateral, pointed at the tip, 5 to 11 centimeters in length, and with toothed margins. The leaves are aromatic when crushed. The flowers are greenish white, fragrant, about 8 millimeters in diameter, and are borne in panicles which are 15 to 20 centimeters long.

This species is a native of the Philippines, is widely distributed, and is abundant in some places. It is occasionally cultivated.

Genus TODDALIA

TODDALIA ASIATICA (L.) Kurz.

Local names: *Atáñgen, bugkáu, bukkáu, subit* (Benguet) ; *dauág* (Rizal).

TODDALIA ASIATICA OIL

According to D. Hooper,† the oil obtained by distilling the leaves of this species has a pleasant odor resembling verbena or basilicum. Gildemeister and Hoffman ‡ state that the oil

---

* Brooks, B. T., New Philippine essential oils. Philippine Journal of Science, Section A, Volume 6 (1911), page 344.

† Schimmel, Semi-annual report (1893).

‡ Die Aetherischen Öle, Berlin (1899), page 601.

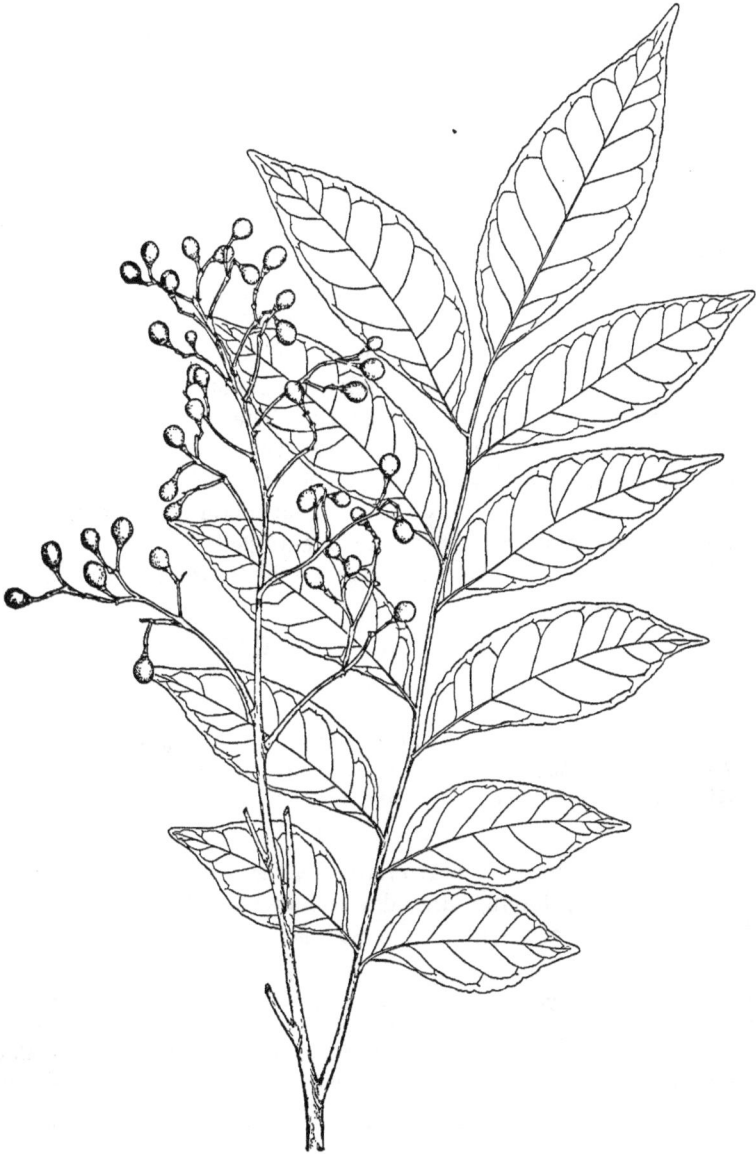

FIGURE 71. CLAUSENA ANISUM-OLENS (KAYUMANIS). $\times\frac{1}{2}$.

is valuable as a low-grade perfume oil. Brooks * says that it is commercially profitable to distill the oil. He reports his investigation as follows:

The leaves yielded 0.08 per cent of oil by steam distillation. On freezing, the oil deposited 18 per cent of a white crystalline, very volatile compound, having an odor closely resembling that of camphor. After recrystallizing the substance twice from petroleum ether, the melting point was 96.5° to 97°. The compound is very unstable. A pure specimen of it changed in 24 hours to a pasty mixture of oil and unchanged crystals. It was not further investigated. The oil had an odor suggesting a mixture of camphor and lemon grass. Its constants were as follows: $N\frac{30°}{D}$, 1.4620; specific gravity, $\frac{30°}{30°}$0.9059.

The oil is largely linaloöl, since the fraction boiling from 195° to 200° yields citral on oxidation with chromic acid mixture.

Toddalia asiatica is a spiny, woody vine. The leaves are alternate and trifoliate. The leaflets are pointed at both ends and 5 to 8 centimeters in length. The flowers are small, greenish, and borne on rather large compound inflorescences. The fruits are small and are borne in fairly large clusters. They are considerably less than a centimeter in diameter and when dry are distinctly three- to five-angled.

This species is common in second-growth forests and is also found in virgin forests.

Family VERBENACEAE

Genus LANTANA

LANTANA CAMARA L.   LANTÁNA.

Local names: *Albahaca de caballo* (Spanish in Zamboanga); *bahug-bahug* (Negros); *boho-boho* (Iloilo); *coronítas* (Manila); *lantána* (Tarlac, Cavite, Batangas, Laguna); *tinta-tintáhan* (Manila).

LANTÁNA OIL

This species has very aromatic leaves from which Bacon † obtained an oil having an odor somewhat like that of sage. Concerning his experiments he writes:

Seventy kilos of the leaves distilled with steam gave 60 cubic centimeters of a light yellow oil; 100 kilos gave 245 cubic centimeters, and 110 kilos gave 78 cubic centimeters of oil.

These results show that the yield of oil evidently varies considerably, the differences depending upon the season, age of the leaves, etc. The oil has a specific gravity of $\frac{30°}{4°}=0.9132$; $N\frac{30°}{D}=1.4913$; $A\frac{30°}{D}=+11.5$. Its

---

* Brooks, B. T., New Philippine essential oils. Philippine Journal of ⟨ Science, Section A, Volume 6 (1911), page 333.

† Bacon, R. F., Philippine terpenes and essential oils, III. Philippine Journal of Science, Section A, Volume 4 (1909), page 127.

'odor reminds me somewhat of sage. Fifty grams distilled *in vacuo* gave two fractions as follows:

(1) Twenty-two grams boiling between 125° to 130° at 12 millimeters $N\frac{30°}{D} = 1.4892$.

(2) Twenty-four grams boiling between 130° and 140° at 11 millimeters; $N\frac{30°}{D} = 1.4970$.

If on further investigation this oil proves to be of any value, the cultivation of the plant is certainly a commercial possibility.

Lantana camara is an erect or half-climbing, hairy, aromatic shrub, usually 1 to 2 meters in height when erect, and higher when climbing. The leaves are rounded at the base and pointed at the tip, with toothed margins, and are from 5 to 10 centimeters in length. The flowers are pink, red, or yellow, and are borne in many-flowered heads. The fruit is a small, almost black berry.

This species grows abundantly and luxuriantly and is common in the waste places of the Philippines. It is a native of tropical America.

Family LABIATAE

Genus OCIMUM

OCIMUM BASILICUM L.   Balanói or Sweet Basil.

Local names: *Albaháca* (Spanish); *balanái* (Rizal); *balanói* (Batanes Islands, Tayabas); *bauing, solási* (Balabac Island); *bidái* (Union); *kalu-ui* (Basilan); *kamáñgi* (Culion Island).

SWEET BASIL OIL

Watt * says that:

"The whole plant has an aromatic odor, which is improved by drying. Its taste is aromatic and somewhat cooling and saline." (*Pharmacog. Ind.*) The seeds, which are much used medicinally in some parts of India, are small, black, oblong (one-sixteenth inch long), slightly arched on one side and flattened on the other, blunt pointed. They have no odor, but an oily, slightly pungent taste. When placed in water they become coated with a semi-transparent mucilage. Steeped in water, they form a mucilaginous jelly (*U. C. Dutt, Murray, Dymock, &c.*). Their properties are said to be demulcent, stimulant, diuretic, and diaphoretic. * * * The plant has a strong aromatic flavor like that of cloves and is often used for culinary purposes as a seasoning. The seeds are sometimes steeped in water and eaten. They are said to be cooling and very nourishing. In Kanawar they are sometimes eaten mixed in ordinary bread (*Stewart, Pb. Pl.*). They are largely employed, especially by the Mohammedans of Eastern Bengal, infused in water, to form a refreshing and cooling drink.

When the herb *Ocimum basilicum* is distilled it yields sweet

---

* Watt, G., Dictionary of the economic products of India. Volume 5 (1891), page 441.

basil oil, which is a yellowish-green, volatile oil lighter than water. Parry * states that it has an excellent fragrance and is used in making mignonette extract. The yield of oil obtained from the herb is about 1.5 per cent or less.

Ocimum basilicum is an erect, branched under-shrub 0.5 to 1.5 meters in height. It is smooth, or somewhat hairy, and very aromatic. The leaves are entire or slightly toothed and 1.5 to 3 centimeters long. The flowers are borne in racemes which are 8 to 15 centimeters long. The corolla is pink or purplish and 9 to 10 millimeters long.

This species is apparently common and widely distributed from the Batanes Islands to southern Mindanao.

Genus OCIMUM

OCIMUM SANCTUM L.   Sulási or Holy Basil.

Local names: *Albaháca* † (Spanish); *balanói* (Tagalog); *bidái* (Iloko); *kolokogo* (Tayabas); *kalúi* (Basilan); *kamáñgi* (Bisaya); *katigau* (Misamis); *kamangkáu* (Camarines); *lokolokó* (Polillo); *magau* (Cotabato); *sulási* (Tagalog).

HOLY BASIL OIL

This species, known as holy basil or tulsí, is the sacred plant of India.

Watt ‡ states that:

The *Tulsí* is the most sacred plant in the Hindu religion; it is consequently found in or near almost every Hindu house throughout India.◦ Hindu poets say that it protects from misfortune and sanctifies and guides to heaven all who cultivate it. * * * Under favourable circumstances, it grows to a considerable size, and furnishes a woody stem large enough to make beads for the rosaries used by Hindus on which they count the number of recitations of their deity's name.

According to Bacon § 13.86 kilos of leaves which were forty-eight hours old at the time of distillation gave 83.3 grams of a green-colored oil (0.6 per cent). This oil had a sweet, anise-like odor and the following properties:—Refractive index, $N\frac{30°}{D}$ $=1.5070$; optical rotation, $A\frac{30°}{D}=0$; specific gravity, $\frac{30}{30°}$ $=0.952$; saponification number, 2.8.

---

* Parry, E. J., Chemistry of essential oils and artificial perfumes, page 308.

† This name belongs properly to the preceding species.

‡ Watt, G., Dictionary of the economic products of India, Volume 5 (1891), page 444.

§ Bacon, R. F., Philippine terpenes and essential oils, IV. **Philippine Journal of Science**, Section A, Volume 5 (1910), page 261.

The oil consists to a large extent of methyl homoanisic acid, melting at 85°, being obtained by oxidizing the fraction boiling from 85° to 95° at 9 millimeters pressure. Bacon also states that 65 small plants gave 2.5 kilos of fresh leaves, which when steamed-distilled gave 32 grams of oil.

Ocimum sanctum is an erect, herbaceous or half-woody, coarse plant, 1 meter or less in height. The stems and younger parts of the plant are covered with spreading hairs. The leaves are opposite, pointed at the tip, somewhat rounded or pointed at the base, 2 to 4 centimeters long, and with toothed margins. The flowers are about 7 millimeters long and pink.

This species is cultivated for its fragrant leaves and is occasionally spontaneous in waste places. It is found throughout the Philippines, but is certainly not a native of the Archipelago.

Genus POGOSTEMON

POGOSTEMON CABLIN Benth. (Fig. 72).   PATCHOULI or KABLÍN.

Local names: *Kabilíng* (Pampanga); *kablín* (Ilocos Sur, Abra, Bontók, Tagalog provinces); *kabling* (Ilocos Sur, Bulacan, Laguna, Mindoro); *kadlín* (Batangas); *kadling* (Rizal); *kadlóm* or *kadlúm* (Tagalog provinces, Camarines, Albay, Sorsogon, Leyte); *sárok* (Igorot).

PATCHOULI OIL

The species *Pogostemon cablin* is highly valued for the perfume oil, patchouli, obtained from its leaves. The dried leaves, which are very fragrant, are sometimes used for scenting wardrobes. It is said that they prevent the clothes from being attacked by moths. Patchouli is a common perfume in India and China, and goods, such as shawls, exported from these countries owe their peculiar odor to the patchouli plant.

The dried leaves of *Pogostemon cablin*, when distilled, yield about 3.5 per cent of patchouli oil, which is used in making perfumes and scented soaps. Formerly patchouli oil was considered a very high-grade perfume base, but it is now more frequently used in lower grades. The pure oil has a strong musky odor and is mixed with other essential oils in making perfumes.

According to Mann,* the etheral oil is present in small quantities in the fresh leaves, and only develops through a kind of fermentation of the cut leaves packed into bundles. This explains why the yield from the dried leaves is about 3.5 to 4 per cent, while from fresh leaves it is much less. Mann says that the pronounced patchouli scent is only popular in a very few cases, like the export business to tropical countries. However, the oil serves many purposes in perfumery, giving a fine

---

* Mann, H., The American Perfumer, Volume 8 (1913–1914), page 144.

shade to various combinations without being obtrusive. It is therefore valuable as a so-called fixing agent. It is used with otto of roses, jasmine, cassia, fine musk and labdanum. For cheaper qualities of patchouli perfumes, benzylacetate is a very good material; it aids in dissipating the severe patchouli odor and for this reason is frequently utilized. With very cheap articles, oil of cloves and also artificial musk are employed. The scent is used with good results to combat the frequently very obtrusive odor of perspiration, completely suppressing it. Mann says:

Besides patchouli perfumes, patchouli toilet water also is used. This is especially popular with the harem ladies of Turkish and Arabic Pashas, who pay enormous prices for fine qualities. These toilet waters are worked with infusion of jasmine, but there are also some to be found in trade containing menthol, which gives an odd shade, and is very well liked. Otto of roses also is added and so is some fine kananga oil, all in combination with the finest patchouli oil, thus preventing its domination.

Askinson * gives the following formulas for patchouli perfumes:

Essence of patchouli

Oil of patchouly	ounces....	1½
Oil of rose	do.........	⅜
Alcohol	quarts....	5

Extract of patchouli

Extract of orange flower	quart....	1
Oil of patchouly	ounces....	1½
Oil of rose	grains....	150
Alcohol	gallon....	1

Patchouli powder

Patchouly herb	pounds....	2
Oil of patchouly	grains....	30
Musk	do.........	15

The constants of patchouli oil obtained from different countries vary considerably. This is shown by the figures in Table 35 which are quoted by Parry.†

TABLE 35.—*Constants of patchouli oil.*

Constants.	Java plants.	Singapore plants.
Specific gravity	0.922 at 25°	0.949 at 25°
Optical rotation	—16° 10′	—58° 24′
Initial boiling point	130°	230°
Distils between 250°—270°	50 per cent.	60 per cent.

* Askinson, G. W., Perfumes and cosmetics, (1915).

† Parry, E. J., The chemistry of essential oils and artificial perfumes, (1908).

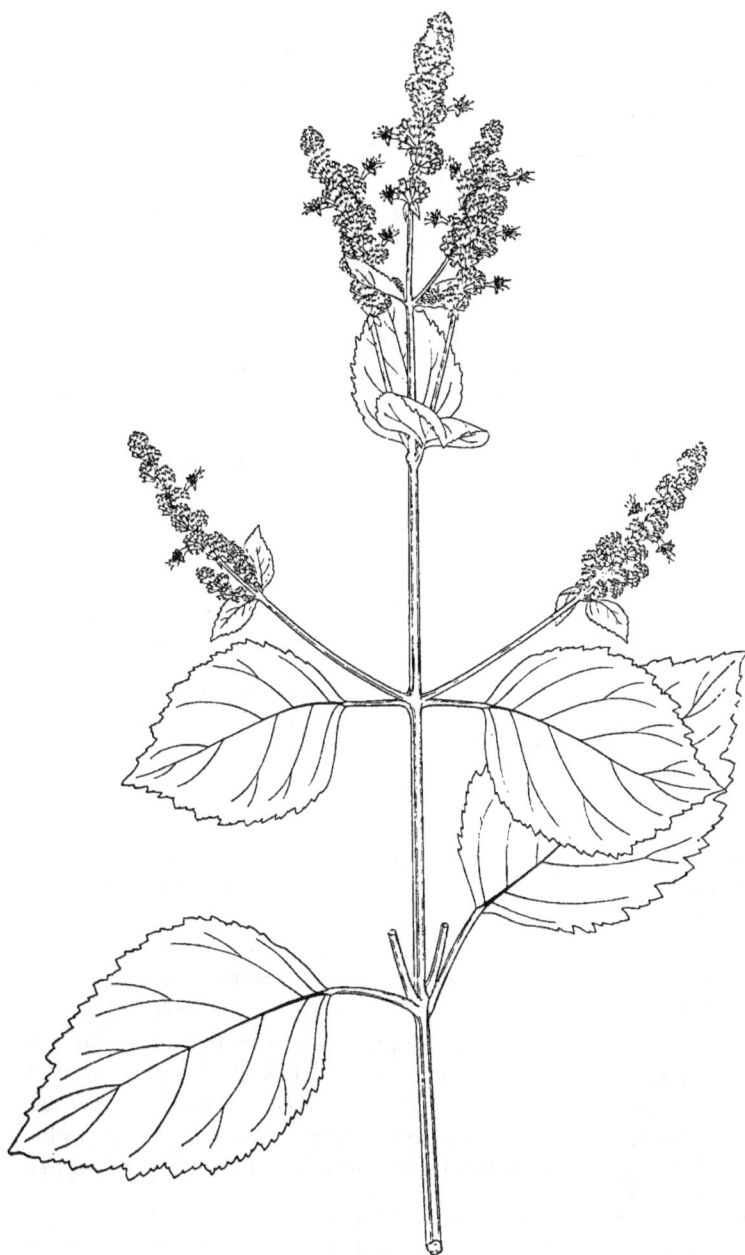

FIGURE 72. POGOSTEMON CABLIN (PATCHOULI OR KABLÍN), THE SOURCE OF PATCHOULI OIL. ×⅓.

According to Gildermeister–Kremers * patchouli alcohol, $C_{15}H_{26}O$, is an odorless constituent of patchouli oil, from which it separates in crystals that melt at 56°.

Pogostemon cablin is an erect, branched, hairy herb .5 to 1 meter in height. It is aromatic when crushed. The leaves are opposite, pointed at the tip, and usually obtusely pointed at the broad base. The margins are coarsely and doubly toothed. The flowers are borne in terminal and axillary spikes which are 2 to 8 centimeters long and 1 to 2.5 centimeters in diameter. The corolla is pink-purple and 8 millimeters long.

This species is found throughout the Philippines in cultivation and is also wild. There seems to be a great deal of uncertainty as to the original home of *Pogostemon cablin*. It is cultivated in many parts of the Indo-Malayan region, but apparently rarely, if ever, flowers in India, Ceylon, Singapore, and Java. It appears to produce flowers freely only in the Philippines.

Family COMPOSITAE

Genus BLUMEA

BLUMEA BALSAMIFERA DC. (Fig. 73).   SAMBÓNG.

Local names: *Alibhón* (Negros); *alimón* (Negros); *bukadkád* (Samar); *kalibón* (Cuyo Islands); *kalibura* (Palawan); *lakadbúlan* (Camarines); *sambón* (Zamboanga); *sambóng* (Tarlac, Bataan, Bulacan, Manila, Palawan, Laguna, Mindoro, Basilan, Tayabas, Zambales, Batangas, Rizal, Balabac Island, Misamis); *sobósob* (Ilocos Norte and Sur, Abra, Pangasinan); *takamain* (Davao).

SAMBÓNG OIL

The leaves of *Blumea balsamifera* are used locally for poisoning fishes, and medicinally for a number of purposes. The roots are also utilized medicinally.

Bacon † distilled the leaves of this plant and obtained a yield of from 0.1 to 0.4 per cent of a yellow oil with a camphor-like odor. This oil was almost pure l-borneol. As this substance readily oxidizes to camphor, the oil, according to Bacon, should be valued at from one-half to three-fourths of the price of the camphor. Bacon estimates that the leaves could be cut four times a year. According to some experiments made in Indo-China, ‡ it is possible to obtain 50,000 kilos of leaves per hectare

---

* Gildermeister, E. and Kremers, E., The volatile oils, (1913).

† Bacon, R. F., Philippine terpenes and essential oils, III. Philippine Journal of Science, Section A, Volume 4 (1909), page 127.

‡ Lan, M. M., Camphus du Tonkin. Bulletin Economique, Gouvernement General de L'indo-Chine. New Series Volume 9 (1907), page 192.

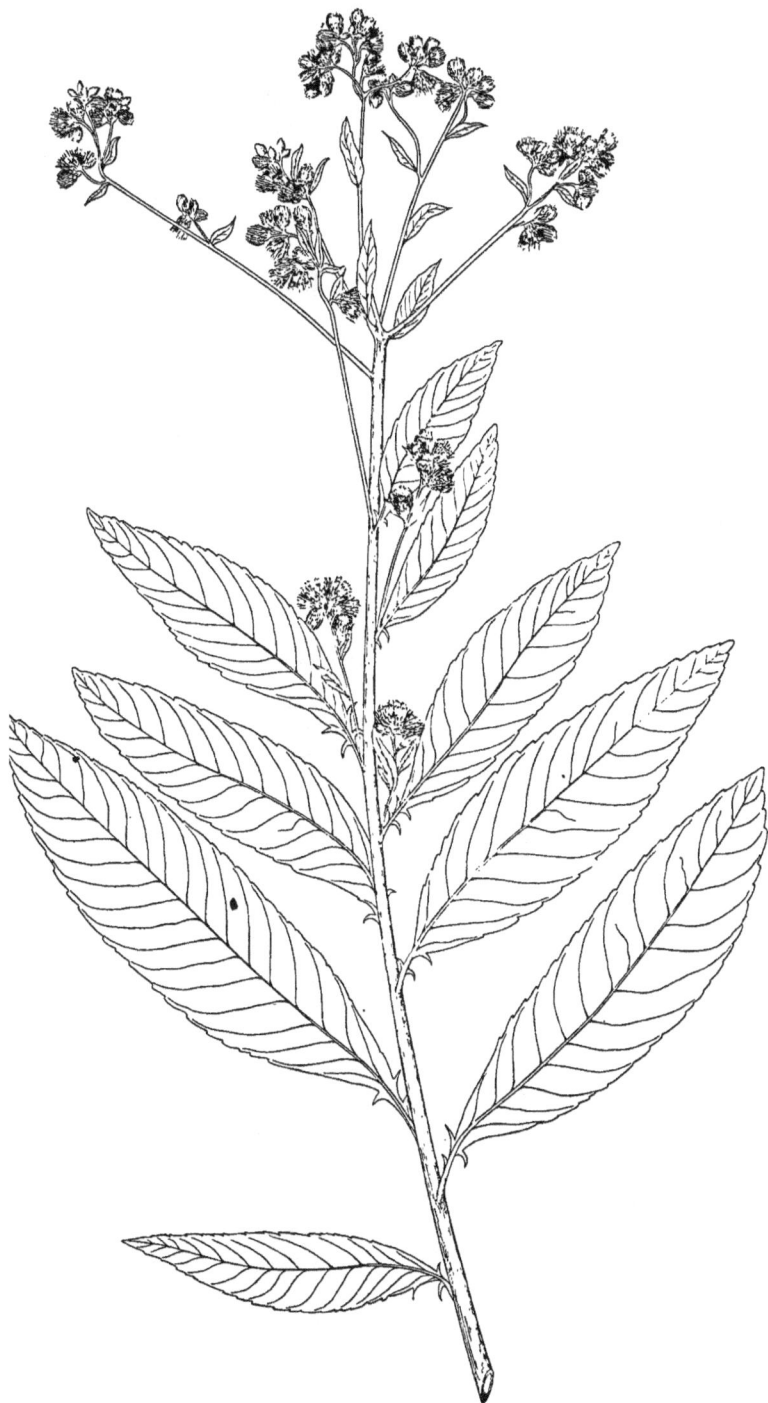

FIGURE 73. BLUMEA BALSAMIFERA (SAMBÓNG), A SOURCE OF CAMPHOR. X⅓.

per year, which would give a possible borneol yield of from 50 to 200 kilos per hectare.   Although this plant grows vigorously in the Philippines, it is questionable if it could be cultivated profitably.

Blumea balsamifera is a coarse, erect, half-woody herb 1.5 to 3 meters in height.   The stems are 2.5 centimeters in diameter.   The leaves are from 7 to 20 centimeters in length, spear shaped, and with toothed margins and short petioles.

This species grows very abundantly in waste places in the Philippines.   It is frequently found in grass areas, as it readily sprouts from the ground after the aerial parts of the plant have been killed by fire.   It is thus one of the comparatively few species of plants which can withstand grass fires.

INDEX

www.ingramcontent.com/pod-product-compliance
Lightning Source LLC
Chambersburg PA
CBHW020530270326
41927CB00006B/521